j616.2   Silverstein, Alvin.
SIL
          Common cold and flu.

$17.95   03/18/1995

DATE			

—Diseases and People—

COMMON COLD AND FLU

Alvin, Virginia, and Robert
Silverstein

ENSLOW PUBLISHERS, INC.

Bloy St. and Ramsey Ave.   P.O. Box 38
Box 777   Aldershot
Hillside, N.J. 07205   Hants GU12 6BP
U.S.A.   U.K.

For Matthew R. Nunn—
a wonderful addition to our family

Library of Congress Cataloging-in-Publication Data

Silverstein, Alvin.
    Common cold and flu / Alvin, Virginia, and Robert Silverstein.
        p. cm. — (Diseases and people)
    Includes bibliographical references and index.
    Summary: Describes the history, causes, prevention, and treatment
of the common cold and flu, as well as the effects on people and society.
    ISBN 0-89490-463-9
    1. Cold (Disease)—Juvenile literature. 2. Influenza—Juvenile literature. [1. Cold
(Disease) 2. Influenza.] I. Silverstein, Virginia. II. Silverstein, Robert. III. Title. IV.
Series.
RF361.S55 1994
616.2'05—dc20   93-4685
                                                    CIP
                                                        AC

Printed in the United States of America

10 9 8 7 6 5 4 3 2

Illustration Credits:
Bob Husth, pp. 51, 55, 66; Bruce D. Korant, Ph.D. and John T. Stasny, Ph.D., p.
21; Centers for Disease Control, p. 80 (top and bottom); David Umberger, Purdue
University, p. 98; Elliot C. Dick, Ph.D., University of Wisconsin-Madison
Medical School, p. 38; National Archives, p. 73; Smithsonian Institution, p. 47;
UPI/Bettmann, pp. 25, 31, 76, 89.

Cover Illustration: © Yoav Levy / Phototake NYC

Contents

Acknowledgments

The authors are very grateful to Lynnett Brammer, Public Health Scientist at the Influenza Branch, Centers for Disease Control, and Drs. Mary Ann LoFrumento and Fern Gotfried of Morristown Memorial Hospital for their careful reading of the manuscript and their many helpful comments and suggestions.

Thanks also to Dr. Elliot C. Dick of the University of Wisconsin for his generous help, and to all the others who have kindly supplied information and photographs. Special thanks to Bob Husth and his family, who helped to dramatize vividly the trials of cold sufferers.

THE COMMON COLD

What is it? An infectious disease caused by one of about 200 cold viruses; affects the upper respiratory tract.

Who gets it? All ages (most common in children), all races, both sexes.

How do you get it? By touching virus-contaminated people or things, then touching one's eyes or nose; or by breathing air that contains virus-contaminated droplets.

What are the symptoms? Scratchy throat, runny nose, congestion, sneezing, watery/itchy eyes, cough, hoarseness, tiredness, reduced sense of smell and taste; fever (in children).

How is it treated? Rest, drinking plenty of fluids, keeping warm; over-the-counter medications for symptoms (decongestants, cough medicines).

How can it be prevented? Avoiding close contact with people with colds or with things they have touched; washing hands regularly; maintaining good general resistance by sensible eating, exercise, and cleanliness; using experimental paper tissues treated with virus-killing chemicals could help prevent spread.

Common Miseries

The *Apollo 9* mission was nearly ready to take off on an orbital flight in February 1969 when the countdown was suddenly interrupted and the flight was delayed. The reason: All three astronauts on the crew were suffering with stuffed-up noses, sore throats, and fatigue. They hadn't fallen victim to an exotic "space bug"—they just had colds. The launch had to be delayed for a full week, until the astronauts recovered. NASA officials estimated that the delay cost about $500,000, and the media talked about "the world's most expensive cold."[1] Subsequently, NASA took care to isolate space crews before scheduled launches to avoid another round of costly colds. But in 1990 it happened again. Blast-off of the space shuttle *Atlantis* was delayed for a week, mainly because crew commander John Creighton had a cold and was too congested to fly. This cold cost NASA $2.7 million.[2]

Almost everyone knows what it feels like to have a cold. In fact, most people can expect to have fifty to one hundred colds during their lifetimes.[3] The chances are that one out of every twenty people reading this book has a cold right now, and almost one out of three has had a cold in the past two weeks![4]

The common cold is the world's most common illness. But that's really the only common thing about it. One person's cold might not be anything like another's, and the cold you have now may not feel at all like the one you'll have six months from now. Sometimes it's even hard to tell whether what you really have is a cold, allergies, the flu, or something else. They may all have similar symptoms, such as a stuffed-up, runny nose, watery eyes, coughs, sneezes, and headaches; but their causes are quite different.

People have been having colds probably since prehistoric times. But until the last hundred years or so, no one really understood what caused them. Scientists today know a lot about colds. In spite of the tremendous progress we have made toward treating and curing many different diseases, though, there is no cure for the common cold.

The common cold is not a life-threatening illness. Compared to many other diseases, colds are not usually very serious. Most people get over them in about a week. But colds make us feel miserable—and they take their toll on society, too. Collectively, Americans suffer about a billion colds a year.[5] More people miss school and work because of colds than from all other illnesses combined, and the lost working time costs society billions of dollars. The cost of colds is high for individuals, too: Each year Americans spend five billion dollars on doctor's visits and medicines to treat colds.[6]

Influenza, or "the flu," is an illness that is very similar to the common cold. But the flu usually feels a lot worse. It is also a much more dangerous illness. It makes the body so weak that some people become susceptible to other serious illnesses, such as bronchitis or pneumonia. The very young and the elderly are especially vulnerable. In a typical year more than ten thousand Americans die from flu complications, and pneumonia and influenza together are currently the sixth leading cause of death in the United States.[7]

The flu is a very contagious illness, and it seems to spread quickly each year during the winter "flu season," usually affecting from 10 to 50 percent of the nation. Every ten years or so, the flu sweeps across the whole world.

Scientists have made great leaps in understanding the common cold and influenza in the past decade. As researchers study these common ailments, they are gaining knowledge that someday may cure them, but they are also discovering information that will be useful in curing other more serious illnesses, too.

This book will discuss these two respiratory diseases, first colds and then the flu, describing their causes and symptoms, suggesting how they can be treated and prevented, and evaluating their impact on our world.

2

Colds and Flu Through the Ages

The ancient Greek physician Hippocrates had a theory about what caused colds. Nearly 2,400 years ago, he suggested that the miserable stuffed-up feeling was the result of too much waste matter building up in the brain. He claimed that a runny nose, one of the most typical cold symptoms, was simply an overflowing of this waste matter.

In the Middle Ages most people looked to superstitions for the explanations of things that happened to them. Illnesses were believed to be caused by demons and other evil influences. Sneezing was considered particularly dangerous, because a person's soul might escape from the body during the sneeze, and a demon might sneak in to replace it. Covering one's mouth while sneezing was thought to help keep the soul inside.

After the Renaissance, doctors began to learn more about how the body works, and scientific explanations for sickness became more widely accepted. Some of them sound rather fanciful today. Seventeenth-century Italians, for example, believed that influenza was caused by the influence of the stars, because the flu always seemed to occur at a particular time of year. (In fact, that is how influenza got its name—it is the Italian word for "influence.")

Through the ages, one of the most popular beliefs has been that colds come from being exposed to cold weather, because many people get colds when it's cold outside. One man who did not agree with the popular idea that colds are the result of getting wet and chilled was Benjamin Franklin, the eighteenth-century

WHAT DO YOU SAY TO A SNEEZE?

Our custom of saying "God bless you!" when someone sneezes dates back to medieval times. It was intended to ward off demons that might slip into the sneezer's open mouth. Customs differ in other countries, though. A German would answer a sneeze with a quick *"Gesundheit!"* meaning "Good Health!" In French the polite response is *"A vos souhaits,"* which roughly means "May your wishes come true."

statesman and inventor. He pointed out that he went swimming in the river every evening for two or three hours and never caught a cold. Franklin believed that colds were caused by substances in people's sweat and breath, carried to others by the air. So, he claimed, breathing plenty of fresh air would help prevent colds.

Discoveries in the Microworld

For centuries some scientists had suspected that many illnesses were caused by tiny infectious particles, too small to see. In 1683 Dutch scientist Antonie van Leeuwenhoek was the first to observe tiny living creatures called bacteria with a microscope that he invented. In the 1870s Louis Pasteur proved that milk that was contaminated with a particular type of bacteria caused a disease called tuberculosis. Many scientists began to believe that all contagious illnesses were caused by bacteria.

In 1898, though, a Dutch botanist named Martinus Willem Beijerinck questioned this belief. He conducted experiments with tobacco leaves that were infected with tobacco mosaic disease, which causes blotchy spots on the leaves. Beijerinck concluded that the disease was caused by something smaller than a bacterium.

The tiny germ that was responsible for the tobacco disease came to be called a virus, from a Latin word meaning "a slimy liquid" or "a poisonous substance." Since these tiny viruses could not be grown under the normal laboratory conditions that scientists used for growing bacteria, the Dutch researcher reasoned that in order for a virus to reproduce it "must be incorporated into the living cytoplasm of the cell, into whose multiplication it is, as it were, passively drawn."[1]

In 1901 yellow fever became the first disease in humans that was linked to a virus. Scientists now know of hundreds of viral diseases, such as the common cold and the flu.

Do Viruses Cause Colds?

A German scientist named Walter von Kruse was one of the first to suggest that viruses cause colds. In 1914 he took nasal secretions from the noses of cold sufferers. He filtered the material so that there were no bacteria present. Then he placed several drops of the filtered material into the noses of healthy volunteers, and, sure enough, they caught colds. But most scientists were not convinced by von Kruse's findings until they were confirmed in 1938 by Alphonse R. Dochez, an American microbiologist.

During the 1930s Wade H. Frost, the first dean of public health at Johns Hopkins University in Baltimore, carefully analyzed where and when colds occurred. He found that they occurred in clusters of small outbreaks, but that there was no way to predict when they would occur or how severe they would be. In 1941 Frost concluded that colds must be caused by many different microorganisms. But no one had yet identified those microorganisms.

Scientists took several steps toward discovering what really causes colds in the next few decades. In 1939 the electron microscope was developed, and researchers could finally see viruses.

In 1949 John Enders of the Boston Children's Hospital figured out a way to grow viruses in the laboratory. This made it much easier to isolate viruses so that they could be identified. It also paved the way for other virus researchers, such as Jonas Salk and Albert Sabin, who developed vaccines against the poliovirus that causes polio. In 1954 Enders received a Nobel Prize in Medicine for his achievement.

Finally, in 1955, Sir Christopher Andrewes, who founded the Common Cold Research Unit in Salisbury, England, identified a virus that caused colds. Polio had been "wiped out" with the development of a vaccine that protected people from the virus that caused it. Some people believed that now that a cold virus had been identified, a vaccine against the common cold would soon be developed. Unfortunately, it was not long before scientists discovered other viruses that also cause colds, and by the 1980s more than two hundred cold-causing viruses had been identified. Most vaccines can protect against only one type of virus or bacteria. Creating a vaccine that can provide protection against more than two hundred different viruses will be quite a feat.

Who Gets Colds?

People all around the world catch colds. Surprisingly, those who live in tropical climates have almost as many colds as we do in the United States. And people who live in the coldest climates, such as the Arctic, actually get the fewest colds!

Colds can strike people of all ages, but children get them most frequently. A baby can expect to have six to nine colds before his or her first birthday.[3] Before the age of four, boys catch more colds than girls, but from four onward girls catch

14

more.[4] As we get older we generally get fewer colds. The elderly get the least, often barely averaging one cold per year. Parents and teachers have a lot of contact with children, so it's not surprising that they catch more colds than adults who have no children. Young women have more colds than men, probably because women usually spend more time with children.[5] For some unexplained reason, one out of twenty people will never experience a cold!

Why Do Children Get the Most Colds?

"Starting at about age six months children lose the immunity they received from their parents," says Carlo Tabellario, a

THE "COLD SEASON"

People can get colds at any time of year, but here in the northern hemisphere they are most common in the winter. Tropical countries have no winter season, but they do have a "cold season," colds are most common there during the rainy season. On the Caribbean island of Trinidad, for example, colds are at their peak in June and July. That's when people are crowded indoors and colds have a better chance to spread.

pediatrician at Torrance Memorial Medical Center in California. "From this point they begin developing their own immunity. That's one reason they have more colds. Beyond the age of three years, however, the frequency of colds begins to slow down."[6]

Another reason children get more colds is that they spend more time in closer contact with one another than adults do. For example, in day-care centers, the chances are that at any particular time one out of four children will have a cold.[7] Colds are contagious. They spread from one person to another. Children touch each other more than adults, and they are also less likely to cover their mouths when coughing and sneezing.

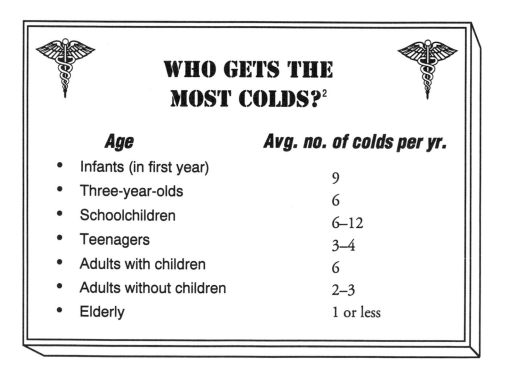

WHO GETS THE MOST COLDS?[2]

Age	Avg. no. of colds per yr.
• Infants (in first year)	9
• Three-year-olds	6
• Schoolchildren	6–12
• Teenagers	3–4
• Adults with children	6
• Adults without children	2–3
• Elderly	1 or less

What Is a Cold?

Through much of the 1992 presidential campaign, Bill Clinton was fighting a stuffy nose and a sore, scratchy throat. The millions of Americans who watched or listened to the first candidates' debate could hear the hoarseness of his voice. Finally, on the Sunday before the election, Clinton lost his voice completely and his wife had to finish the speech he had begun. He didn't have a cold, though; his symptoms were caused by allergies. A few months later, in a major address shortly after Clinton became President of the United States, listeners noticed the hoarseness again. This time there was a different explanation: The President had a cold.[1]

When Is a Cold a Cold?

Colds cause symptoms that are similar to many other illnesses. So, what is a cold? Doctors use the term "common cold" for upper respiratory infections (that is, ones that affect the breathing passages from the nose to the back of the upper throat and voice box) that are caused by viruses and typically produce a stuffed-up, runny nose and a mild sore throat. (No viruses are involved in allergies, which may produce similar symptoms as the body responds mistakenly to something in the environment, such as plant pollens in the air.)

Bad colds are sometimes called "the flu," but the real flu (influenza) is caused by a different group of germs. Sometimes people make a distinction between a head cold and a chest cold. Actually, infections that involve the lungs are not simple colds but more serious infections.

A Cold by Any Other Name Is Still a Cold

Doctors sometimes call colds acute *coryza,* from the Greek *koryza,* which means "nasal mucus," or *catarrh* from the Greek *katarrhein,* which means "to flow down." Other names include *rhinitis* for inflammation of the nose and *pharyngitis* when the upper throat or pharynx is affected.

My Cold Is Different From Your Cold

By the time we feel a cold "coming on," it has already arrived. There is an 18- to 48-hour incubation period between infection with cold germs and the development of symptoms.[2] Colds often start off with a runny nose or a scratchy throat, then other symptoms may develop. Cold symptoms peak after a few days and then get better until they are gone in a week or two.

However, colds are not the same in different age groups. A large study of four hundred elderly people found that the elderly may have fewer colds but they often last longer. Symptoms lasted from two to forty-six days and many persisted for two to three weeks.[3]

Cold are different for children, too. Adults don't usually run a fever with a cold. "Children run a fever more readily, although not usually more than 102 degrees Fahrenheit. The eyes are itchy. Infants tend to get mild diarrhea. Younger children can have headaches, generalized aches and pains, and a hacking cough, particularly at night," says Angel Cadiz, a Coral Springs, Florida, pediatrician.[4] "Although they get colds more frequently, they are generally probably not as sick as adults when they do get them," comments Howard A. Silverman, an Allentown, Pennsylvania, family physician.[5]

What Causes Colds?

Today we know that most infectious diseases are caused by either bacteria or viruses. Bacteria usually consist of only one cell, the bacterium, too small to see without a microscope. But they are complex giants compared to viruses. If a bacterium were the size of an elephant, a virus would be the size of an ant![6] Viruses are a hundred times smaller than bacteria; scientists couldn't see them until the electron microscope was invented.

Some viruses are only 1/100,000 of an inch long, others only a billionth of an inch. Some are shaped like rods, others like many-sided domes. Many viruses look like snowflakes or crystals.

Each individual virus particle has a protective outer protein coat, surrounding a packet of hereditary information, chemically spelled out in the form of nucleic acids. To reproduce, a virus must penetrate into a living cell. There the virus nucleic acid blueprints take over, directing the host cell to manufacture new viruses instead of making its own cell chemicals. The infected cell is thus turned into a sort of slave factory, dedicated to producing viruses. Eventually, the manufactured viruses burst out of the host cell and spread through the body, infecting new cells.

Some viruses can survive for long periods of time outside living cells, in air, water, or even the vacuum of space. But cold viruses are very particular and cannot survive for more than a few hours outside of their normal habitat, in the nose and back of the throat.

About two hundred different viruses can cause colds. They may look different under a microscope, but most of them produce similar symptoms.

At least 30 to 50 percent of colds are caused by rhinoviruses. (*Rhino* comes from the Greek word for "nose.") One hundred cold-causing rhinoviruses have been identified. Rhinoviruses are very small—two hundred million of them could fit on the period at the end of this sentence. These viruses usually cause colds in the fall and late spring.

Coronaviruses cause 10 to 20 percent of all colds, usually in mid- to late winter. These colds often spread in epidemics.

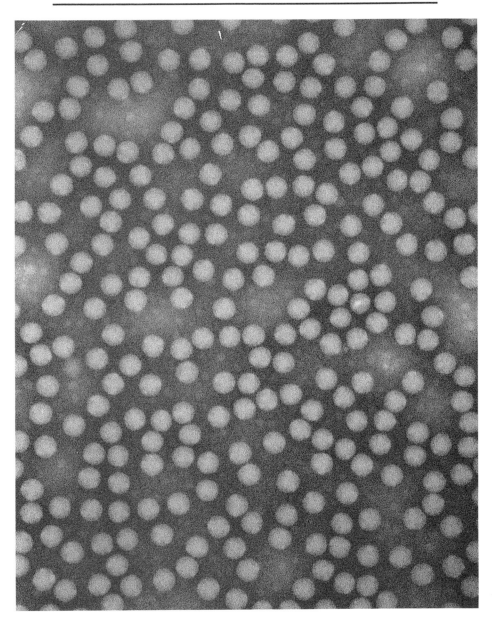

This is one type of human rhinovirus, magnified thousands of times. Over one hundred types of rhinoviruses have been identified.

Adenoviruses may cause spring and summer colds, mainly in children age fifteen or under. Five other families of viruses also contribute to the common cold miseries.

How Cold Viruses Attack Cells

Cold viruses attack cells in the lining of the nose and throat. In order for a virus to get inside a cell, it first has to attach to it. A virus's outer protein coat contains proteins that match up with proteins on the cell membrane of the "host cell" or "target cell" they are attacking. The virus attaches at a special spot on the cell membrane, called a receptor site, into which it fits in just the way a key fits into a lock. The cell receptor becomes the doorway for the virus to enter the cell.

Several hours after cold viruses get into the body, hundreds of thousands of viruses have attached to target cells. A cell will surround the virus in an attempt to destroy the intruder. But this actually works in favor of the virus because it brings the virus inside the cell—just where it was trying to go. The host cell tries to destroy the virus with strong chemicals. But these simply dissolve the virus's outer protein coat, leaving the viral genetic material loose in the cell.

Each healthy cell has its own genetic instruction for producing new cells exactly like itself. It also has the tools to carry this process out (which, of course, viruses don't have). Once the virus's genetic material is free, the nasal cell becomes a slave to the cold virus. The virus substitutes its own genetic instructions for those of the host cell. The virus then tricks the cell into making viruses instead of new host cells.

The first thing the virus does is turn off the cell's reproduction center. Then the virus instructions start the "factory" going again. The host cell first creates virus nucleic acids. Then the outer coats are produced. Finally, the new viruses are put together. Twenty-four hours after the viruses first invaded the cells, one million infected cells have produced ninety million more viruses. The new viruses poke holes in the cell membrane to escape. This ultimately kills the original host cell. The new viruses are now free to infect new cells.

By the second day of a cold, nearly one million nose and throat cells have been killed. These dead cells accumulate, and the body tries to wash them away with a watery fluid in the nose. This is, of course, a runny nose, one of the first cold symptoms. Another early symptom—a scratchy throat—occurs when many of the epithelial cells that line the throat are killed.

Colds are not as serious as many other viral infections because the mucous membrane cells of the upper respiratory system are easily replaced and not as important to the body as other cells are. Influenza viruses can kill more important cells in the lungs, which makes the flu a more serious respiratory infection than a cold.

Body Barriers

Cold germs can get into the body through the nose, through the eyes, or through the mouth. But colds are not as easy to catch as you might think. A single rhinovirus sprayed into the nose of a healthy volunteer causes cold symptoms only 10 to

20 percent of the time.[7] Usually you have to be repeatedly exposed to the same virus strain to become infected, because the body has many barriers to stop invading germs.

Cold viruses that get into the body through the mouth are generally destroyed. Most are swallowed and are sent down to the stomach, where strong digestive juices devour them. Others are swept into the tonsils and adenoids, the throat's garbage disposal units.

Viruses can also get into the body through the eyes. Tears keep our eyeballs moist. Excess tears drain through small ducts from the inside corners of the eyes into the nose. If viruses are rubbed into the eyes, they may be washed down the drainage tubes and end up in the nose.

We usually breathe through our noses, so most cold viruses enter the body this way. There are many protective barriers here, too. First, in the nostrils, several hundred hairs stop dust and tiny water droplets that might be carrying germs.

The body's second line of defense against invading germs is a mucous membrane that lines much of the respiratory tract. Cells in this membrane produce a thick, sticky liquid (mucus) that forms a thin blanket to shield the cells below. Germs are trapped in the sticky mucus. Some membrane cells are equipped with thin hairlike cilia. Millions of them beat back and forth in a wavelike motion, up to 1,000 beats a minute, pushing mucus back up to the mouth where it can be spat out harmlessly, or swallowed. It normally takes from ten to twelve minutes for particles to be moved from the nostrils

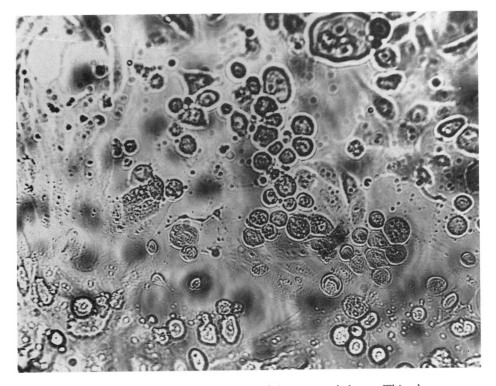

Cold viruses attack cells in the lining of the nose and throat. This photo shows cells that have been affected by the common cold.

to the back of the throat. But tobacco smoke and alcohol may slow down the rate at which the cilia move mucus along. The longer it takes, the greater the chance viruses have to infect cells along the way.

Viruses infect most successfully in cold, dry air. In these conditions the mucus that lines the airway passages can become dried up and less able to carry off invading viruses. But the air that enters the nose is warmed and humidified by a rich supply of blood vessels in the mucous membrane, as it swirls around flaplike structures called turbinates. If you breathe in a quantity of dry air that is 10 degrees Fahrenheit, it will be heated up to 91 degrees with about 75 percent humidity by the time it reaches the top of your throat.[8]

Viruses that make it to the back of the nose or the throat must overcome another barrier. Specialized cells of the immune system use various weapons to fight off viruses and other invaders.

You Can't Always Win the Cold War

If you are generally in good health, your body's defenses may be able to prevent viruses from reaching their targets. But when the defense mechanisms have been weakened by smoking, air pollution, allergies, or another illness, the body may not be able to overcome the viruses' attack. And even healthy people cannot win every cold battle.

You never know that you've been infected with cold germs until they have already caused a lot of damage. Usually you don't even feel those familiar yucky symptoms until two or three days after being infected. By the third day of a cold, symptoms such as runny nose, sneezing, scratchy throat, and coughing are usually very noticeable.

In the 1930s doctors thought that cold symptoms were the result of massive destruction of cells in the nose and throat. But today we know, as Dr. Elliot Dick, a cold expert at the University of Wisconsin, points out, that "the symptoms of a cold are really an immune response."[9] Many of the symptoms of a cold are caused by our own bodies' efforts to fight the virus.

The Body Defends Itself

The immune system is the body's powerful defense against intruders. It coordinates many different types of cells and substances to help fight diseases and protect against future attacks by similar viruses. But it is our own immune system that produces many of a cold's unpleasant symptoms.

The first cells that are attacked by a virus are unable to defend themselves. But several hours before an infected cell releases the new viruses it was ordered to create, a substance called interferon is released into the fluids surrounding the cell. This chemical tells neighboring cells to make an antiviral protein that will fight off viruses. When the virus attacks alerted neighboring cells, they are able to disobey the virus's orders. The warning action of interferon helps delay the spread of infection until the body's big guns can get to the scene.

An hour or so after a virus invasion, cells also give off

LIFE CYCLE OF A COLD

Days 1–3:

Viruses attach to nasal cells, release genetic material, and take over the cells' reproductive machinery, causing cells to create thousands of virus copies.

At first you don't feel anything while all this is going on. But then damaged throat tissues send out chemical alarms that produce inflammation and summon defending white blood cells. Now your throat is sore, and you may have chills and muscle aches.

Days 4–7:

The body's immune system is fighting the viruses, causing symptoms like runny nose, congestion, and watery eyes as the body increases production of fluids to soothe tissues.

Days 7–9:

The immune system gradually wins its battle against the viruses and retains a memory of that particular virus so that it will be able to wipe it out before it can infect cells should it ever get into the body again. Congestion, runny nose, and other cold symptoms gradually disappear.

chemicals such as histamine, bradykinin, and prostaglandins. They prompt cells in the nasal lining to secrete extra mucus, which helps to trap the viruses in the sticky fluid. The chemical messengers also cause inflammation: swelling, pain, heat, and redness around the area of infection. These changes help to slow down virus reproduction, while also making it easier for white blood cells, the body's roving disease fighters, to move around.

The chemicals released by virus-damaged cells also act as distress signals, calling in several kinds of white blood cells. Some, such as macrophages (whose name literally means "big eaters") and neutrophils, gobble down invading germs, destroying them before they can infect cells. Lymphocytes provide more specific defenses. Some are equipped to recognize foreign chemicals, such as the proteins on the outer coat of a virus. Some lymphocytes attack germs directly. Others produce antibodies, proteins that contain mirror images of virus proteins. (The proteins to which antibodies respond are referred to as antigens.) Antibodies attach to viruses, preventing them from attacking their target cells and making them easier for the body's defenders to destroy.

Once you have antibodies protecting you from a particular virus strain, your body will be able to prevent future infections by it—you become immune to it. The antibodies continue to circulate in the blood for years, ready to leap into action against attacks by the same type of virus.

It generally takes about two weeks for the body to make antibodies, so scientists believed these weapons were usually not ready in time to fight a cold or the flu. But antibodies designed to fit one type of virus may also partially block similar viruses. Thus, even if people have never encountered a particular virus, they may already have antibodies that will help to block it.

The various types of white blood cells signal to each other by means of chemicals, which help to identify foreign invaders, summon defenders to the battle, turn loose "killer cells" to attack the invading viruses, help in antibody production, produce fever, and, finally, tell the immune system when the battle is over and it is time to stop fighting.

A Closer Look at Cold Symptoms

Sneezing. When hairs in the nose are tickled by an irritant, such as dust or mucus, nerves are stimulated and provoke a sneeze. The muscles around the lungs contract, causing an explosion of air that shoots particles out as far as twelve feet at speeds of up to one hundred miles an hour. Sneezing helps to get rid of the irritating substance so that it will not pass deeper into the respiratory system.

Coughing. An irritant, such as excess mucus in the upper air passage, causes nerves to trigger a coughing response. The chest and abdominal muscles tighten, and the epiglottis, a flap of tissue at the top of the larynx (the voice box), closes. Pressure builds up inside the larynx as air can't get out. The epiglottis then opens suddenly and all the air bursts out, propelled from the mouth at five hundred miles an hour. Coughing pushes the irritating material up to the back of the

30

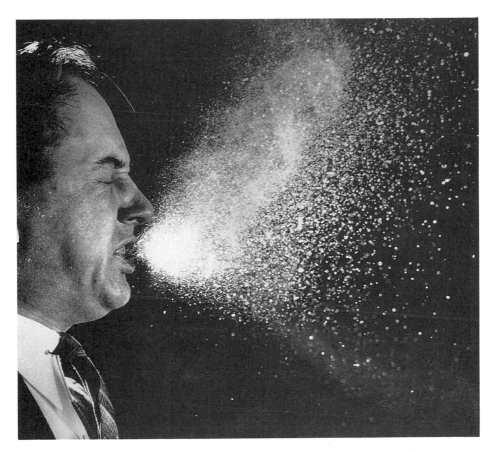

When a person sneezes, he or she releases thousands of particles into the air.
This man's sneeze was captured on film using high-speed photography.

throat so that it can be swallowed or spat out. It is an automatic reaction, but we can also cough voluntarily.

Fever. When you have a fever, everything goes into high gear: Your heart pumps more quickly, breathing speeds up, and you burn food faster than usual. When the body needs to cool down, you break out in a sweat. As the moisture evaporates on the skin's surface it carries heat away. Many experts believe that a mild fever is the body's attempt to kill or disable invading germs and that it can sometimes help us recover from a viral infection.

Runny nose and congestion. These are effects produced by bradykinin and other substances released by virus-damaged cells. The increased fluid in the inflamed tissues makes the

WAR OF THE NOSES

A raw, runny nose is the classic cold symptom. But just what is that runny goop? "It's not all mucus and it's not all leakage from blood vessels. The only word that describes it properly is snot," says cold researcher Jack M. Gwaltney, Jr., head of virology and epidemiology at the University of Virginia.[10]

The fluid that runs out of a runny nose is made up of mucus, dead epithelial cells, dead lymphocytes and other white blood cells, proteins, and viruses. There may also be traces of blood if the nasal lining is irritated. When nasal discharge turns green or yellow researchers say, this usually comes from the accumulation of white blood cells.

mucous membranes swell, which narrows the nasal passages. That is what causes the stuffed-up feeling. The area may become sore when swollen membranes press against nerve endings.

In sinusitis, inflammation has spread to the sinuses (membrane-lined spaces inside the skull bones), which may fill with fluid as the swollen membranes block their drainage. The buildup of pressure may cause headaches. The sinuses normally give the voice resonance during speech and singing; when the sinuses are clogged, the voice sounds flat.

The nasal passages are also connected to the ears, and inflammation may spread to the ear linings. This complication is referred to as otitis and causes the pain of an earache.

Lack of smell. Postage-stamp-sized patches of nerve cells in the nasal membranes normally respond to chemicals in the air and send messages to the brain that are interpreted as smells. When the nose is congested with a cold, these nerves cannot do their job, so we can't smell very well. Taste is closely linked with smell, so foods seem bland when we're sick.

Runny eyes, sore throat. Eyes sometimes become watery because the tear ducts that open into each eye may be infected, too. A scratchy throat is the after-effect of the destruction of cells in the throat's lining. The area becomes dry because the epithelial cells that produce and move the mucus have been killed. Bradykinins also stimulate pain receptors in the throat. Some people get laryngitis when the virus affects the vocal cords in the larynx.

4

How Colds
Are Spread

For nearly half a century, from 1946 to 1990, eighteen thousand people of all ages from all over the world spent unusual vacations in the picturesque countryside around Salisbury, England. A private room, three hot meals a day, and sports such as badminton, table tennis, cricket, and croquet were all free; in addition, the vacationers received £1.75 a day (about $5.00 U.S.) in spending money. All they had to do in return was to try to catch a cold. At the Common Cold Research Unit, dedicated scientists sprayed cold viruses into people's noses and conducted various other experiments to discover just how people catch colds.[1] They and other research groups have found that what "everybody knows" about colds may not necessarily be true.

How Do You Catch a Cold?

Sometimes you have a pretty good idea where you caught a cold—someone close to you may have been sick a day or two ago, for example. But at other times you might not have any idea where you got your cold.

The common cold is a communicable disease—meaning that it is spread from one person to another. Viruses must leave the body of an infected person and get inside the body of a healthy person. The fluids in a cold sufferer's eyes, nose, and throat contain virus particles. The release of viruses from the body is called viral shedding, and it can begin as soon as seven hours after the virus first enters the cells. Viral shedding may continue for weeks after symptoms have disappeared, as well, but the most viruses are shed when colds are at their worst: during the three days following the first sign of symptoms.

The Aerosol-Transmission Theory

Colds are caused by viruses that infect cells in the nose and throat. But how do they get there? After scientists discovered that colds were caused by viruses, it was widely believed that they were carried on droplets that leave the mouth or nose when a sick person coughs, sneezes, or even talks. This is called the aerosol-transmission theory, and it was the view most people held by the turn of the century.

In the 1940s Sir Christopher Andrewes tried to test the aerosol-transmission theory at the Common Cold Research Unit. But many healthy volunteers did not catch colds when he exposed them to coughs and sneezes of cold sufferers. His results greatly challenged the popular view, but scientists were reluctant to give up the idea that colds were spread through the air because it seemed the most obvious way.

Do Hands Spread Colds?

In the 1960s Dr. Jack M. Gwaltney, Jr., and Dr. J. Owen Hendley of the University of Virginia found that there was very little cold virus present in the saliva of cold sufferers.[2] They found it hard to believe that colds were spread by coughing or sneezing saliva droplets. In the 1970s they began to test the theory that most colds were spread through hand-to-hand contact. When fifteen college students rubbed their hands in nasal secretions of people with colds and then touched their eyes or noses, eleven of them caught colds. Only one of twelve students who were seated at a table with coughing and sneezing cold sufferers got sick. Then Gwaltney and Hendley had mothers of children who had colds paint their own hands with virus-killing iodine. These mothers got fewer colds than those who did nothing to their hands.[3]

The researchers also believed that people could catch colds by touching objects that had recently been touched by a cold sufferer. They found that viruses could survive for hours on handkerchiefs, doorknobs, telephones, dishes, books, toys, and other surfaces. Dr. Gwaltney and Dr. Henley concluded that only 10 percent of colds are spread through the air. The rest are spread through touch.[4] You might not think that you touch your eyes and nose very much. But Dr. Gwaltney and Dr. Hendley found in observations that two-thirds of adults and children touched their nose or eyes at least once an hour.[5]

By the early 1980s the medical community had agreed that most colds were probably spread through hand-to-hand contact. But Dr. Elliot Dick of the University of Wisconsin was not convinced. In 1986 he set up an experiment to show that viruses were spread through the air. When healthy subjects played cards with sick ones, 50 to 75 percent of the healthy volunteers came down with colds. Similar results were observed even when the players wore special collars and arm restraints that kept them from touching their faces. "That tells me colds are spread through the air," Dr. Dick says.[6]

Next, the researcher gave healthy volunteers in another group cards and poker chips contaminated by cold viruses to play with. The cards were very gooey, and at first "when they saw those grossly contaminated cards they refused to touch them," say Dr. Dick. But the volunteers did it for science, and not one of them caught a cold! "To me that indicates that it is very hard to transmit a cold by hand," the Wisconsin researcher concludes.[7]

Dr. Dick doesn't believe that colds can be spread by touching contaminated surfaces. "They can be spread by nasal mucus, but once you let it dry, it's almost impossible to spread," he insists.[8]

Testing how colds are spread under laboratory settings could be very different from the way colds travel in the real

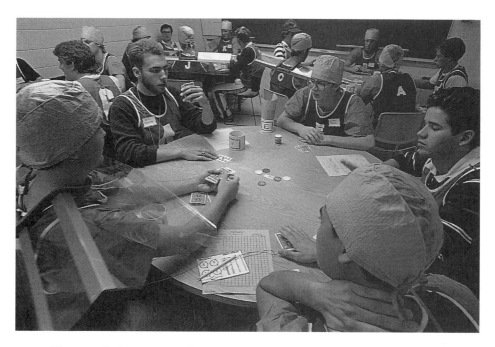

These card players were taking part in a 1986 study by Dr. Elliot Dick to prove that colds are spread through the air.

world. Dr. Gwaltney points out, "We still don't know how colds spread under natural conditions. Dr. Hendley and I have shown they can be transmitted by hand to hand contact. . . . Elliot Dick has established that they can be transmitted by aerosols. It's certainly possible that in the real world, both routes are possible."[9]

Dr. C. Margaret Johnson-Lussenburg at the University of Ottawa has helped make sense of these seemingly contradictory findings. She has found that environmental conditions such as temperature and relative humidity influence which viruses will spread, and which path they will take. Under ordinary conditions of 70°F and 40 percent humidity, rhinoviruses die quickly in aerosol form but survive much better on surfaces. However, in the cooler temperatures and high humidity of early fall and early spring, airborne rhinoviruses thrive, then die off once it gets colder. When the temperature is just above freezing and humidity is high, coronaviruses travel best by air.[11]

Why Do People Get More Colds When It Is Cold Outside?

For centuries people have claimed that getting cold and wet can give you colds. At the Common Cold Unit in England, Sir Christopher Andrewes tested this "chill theory" in 1951. Volunteers were divided into three groups. The first group was given nose drops containing cold viruses and had to stand in wet bathing suits in a cold room for half an hour. The second group was also given viral nose drops but stayed warm and cozy. The members of the third group stood in wet bathing suits in the cold, but were not given the nose drops. Only the volunteers who were exposed to the cold virus came down with colds, and they got them whether they stood in the cold or not. Thus the researchers proved that cold weather does not cause colds.

Nevertheless, people do get more colds in autumn and winter. Researchers believe there are several reasons. School starts in the fall, and children are the major carriers of cold viruses. They spread colds to their parents, who spread them at work, or on buses or trains. During cold weather people

DOES KISSING SPREAD COLDS?

In a University of Wisconsin study, only one out of sixteen student volunteers who kissed a cold-infected student came down with a cold. Other studies have found that it takes one thousand times more rhinovirus to give someone a cold if the virus is dripped on the tongue rather than into the nose. Even a few million rhinoviruses in your mouth will most likely end up destroyed in your stomach or adenoids. On the other hand, adenoviruses (another form of cold virus) can spread orally.[10]

spend most of their time indoors in close contact with other people—ideal conditions for spreading colds by either hand-to-hand contact or aerosol transmission.

Another important factor is that in the winter there is much less humidity in the air, both inside and outside. In dry air nasal mucus tends to dry up and does not cover the nasal cells properly. This gives viruses a better chance to infect the cells below. Nasal cells also produce less immunoglobulin (antibodies) in dry air, so the immune defenses are not as strong.

Studies have shown that if a family member has a cold, other family members have a 40 percent chance of getting it. The greater the contact with a sick person and the more objects the person touches, the greater the risk.

Anyone in poor health, who eats improperly, or who doesn't rest or exercise enough, may be more susceptible to colds. The immune system is weakened when we are not in good health. Chilling, overheating, and exhaustion have also been linked with lower immune defenses.

Cigarette smokers have more severe colds than nonsmokers and have more complications such as bronchitis and pneumonia. Children of parents who smoke tend to have more colds, as well as having other respiratory problems. People who suffer from allergies may also have more severe colds.

Poor people have more colds than wealthy and middle-class people. The reason is that poor people live in more crowded places, have more children, eat poorer diets, and are less able to practice good hygiene.

Don't Worry, Be Happy . . .

An extensive study published in 1991 showed that stress greatly increases a person's chances of catching a cold. "With every increase in psychological stress, there's an increase in the likelihood of developing a cold, given exposure to the virus," says Sheldon Cohen, a professor of psychology at Carnegie-Mellon University in Pittsburgh, who worked with researchers at the Common Cold Unit in England.[14] People under the greatest stress were twice as likely to develop a cold as those

MONDAY BLUES

A classic Michigan cold study found that people come down with colds more on Mondays (the "bluest" day of the week) than on any other day. Is it that we just do not want to go back to school or to work on Mondays? Not necessarily. Remember, colds have an incubation period of a few days. So a cold that develops on Monday was probably caught the previous week after a whole week's worth of contacts with possible cold sufferers at work or school, and the week's stress has worn the body down.[13]

with the least amount of stress when both groups were exposed to cold viruses.

Oddly enough, another study found that people who do not have much contact with friends and neighbors suffer more colds and worse colds than those who have more contact with people. Stress and social isolation may cause a person to be depressed. Studies have found that when people feel sad and hopeless over a period of time, their immune systems are also depressed—levels of immunoglobulin are reduced.

5

Treating A Cold

An old saying claims that if you treat a cold you'll be cured in a week, but if you leave it alone it will go away by itself in seven days. In most cases that old saying is fairly accurate, but few people are willing to just leave a cold alone.

People go to the doctor more for colds than for any other reason. Unfortunately, doctors can't help much to ease a cold sufferer's misery. "Doctors have nothing now that we didn't have ten years ago," says Dr. Arnold Monto, professor of epidemiology and international health at the University of Michigan in Ann Arbor.[1]

Of course, there are plenty of cold remedies that you can buy in the drugstore or supermarket. Medications can make you feel better, but they don't fight the viruses that are causing you to feel sick.

Old Remedies

"A bad cold wouldn't be so annoying if it weren't for the advice of our friends," humorist Kin Hubbard once commented,[2] and people have been suggesting cures for the common cold for a long, long time. Three thousand years ago the Chinese made a tea from a shrub called mahuang to treat a stuffy nose. That folk medicine really worked; the shrub contains the chemical ephedrine, which has a decongestant effect. Pseudoephedrine, a synthetic equivalent, is used in many of today's cold remedies.

In ancient Greece, bloodletting was a popular treatment for colds. The Greeks believed that colds were caused by excess fluid in the body, so a bleeding cut would help the cold sufferer get rid of the excess fluid more quickly. Bloodsucking leeches were also used to suck out fluids.

A milder but similar treatment called "dry cupping" is a traditional folk medicine to cure many ills, still practiced in places such as Greece, Mexico, and Vietnam. Cups are heated and placed on the skin. The hot cups supposedly draw blood away from the diseased organ. Actually, the stinging heat distracts the patients and helps them forget about the cold symptoms. Mustard plaster placed on the skin has a similar effect.

Many other treatments were used to cure colds. The Roman author Pliny advised "kissing the hairy muzzle of a mouse" to cure a cold's coughs and sneezes. Another ancient Roman cure was drinking onion soup. In the twelfth century, the Jewish philosopher and physician Maimonides suggested that chicken soup would help.

Prayer was the treatment suggested by the Catholic church during the Middle Ages. Garlic necklaces and salted herring collars were also recommended, to keep away both colds and evil spirits.

In Colonial America herbal teas and other herbal concoctions were popular. In the 1800s some parents did not bathe their children during the winter because they believed that getting wet in cold weather caused colds. Beards were popular partly because they kept the throat warmer. Many people also turned to "scientific" cold remedies. Pills, potions, powders, and tonics were sold in drugstores and by traveling medicine men. Some remedies were relatively harmless, containing herbs or ingredients such as rum and molasses in the Kickapoo Indian Cure-All. But many popular cure-alls contained strong narcotic drugs such as cocaine, opium, and morphine. Many people became addicted to cough and cold medicines.

All kinds of devices were invented to help cure colds. There were nasal sprays that squirted herbal teas, seawater, or cocaine mixtures into the nostrils. People breathed in vapors from mint leaves or camphorated oil through face masks to relieve congestion. In the early 1900s some doctors even prescribed electric shocks to cure cold symptoms.

In 1830 a German company called Bayer Pharmaceuticals synthesized acetylsalicylic acid. Salicylic acid is a substance found in willow bark, and it has been used since earliest times

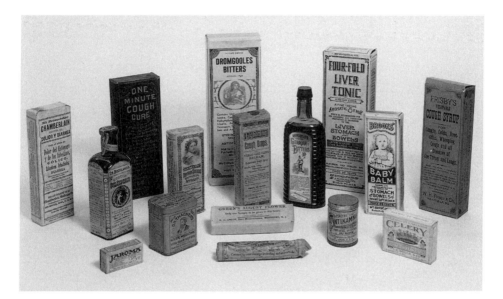

During the 1800s, many types of potions, pills, and tonics were sold to help cure colds and other ailments. While some were harmless, others contained addictive drugs.

as a painkiller. Two thousand years ago, Hippocrates, the father of Greek medicine, recommended chewing willow bark to ease pain; Native Americans also used it to reduce pain and fever. Bayer called its pain reliever aspirin. It became an important tool to relieve cold symptoms such as muscular aches and pains and headaches. Aspirin prevents the production of prostaglandins, body chemicals that cause inflammation. Acetaminophen preparations (such as Tylenol) and ibuprofen (such as Advil) also block prostaglandin production.

In the 1970s scientists linked taking aspirin during flu, chicken pox, or other viral illnesses with Reye's syndrome, a rare but often fatal childhood illness affecting the liver and nervous system. Today, the American Academy of Pediatrics recommends that children and teenagers should take acetaminophen instead of aspirin when they have colds.

Aspirin may not even be a good idea for adults with colds. Since 1975 researchers have reported that aspirin may suppress the immune system and prolong viral shedding. Dr. Neil M. H. Graham, of Johns Hopkins University, points out that doctors are not saying analgesics shouldn't be used for colds, but that "the message is to take them only for the proper symptoms, which are headache and fever."[3]

When To See a Doctor

Americans spend two billion dollars a year going to the doctor for colds, but their expectations are often unrealistic. "People still come in with a cold and ask for a shot of penicillin," says

Dr. Howard A. Silverman, chief of family practice at the Allentown Hospital-Lehigh Hospital Center in Pennsylvania. "But penicillin and other antibiotics do not work for viruses. In fact, to use penicillin or some other antibiotic not only won't work, but could be potentially harmful. In addition to an adverse reaction, bacteria which may cause a secondary infection may become resistant to that antibiotic, causing it to be ineffective."[4]

Sometimes, of course, it is necessary to go to the doctor. Colds can be very serious for babies, elderly people over seventy, pregnant women, and those who suffer from chronic heart or lung conditions. These people should seek a doctor's advice when they come down with a cold.

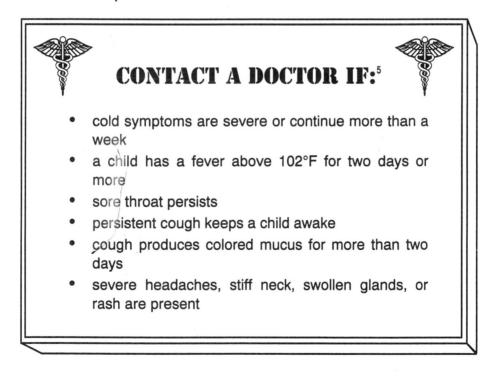

CONTACT A DOCTOR IF:[5]

- cold symptoms are severe or continue more than a week
- a child has a fever above 102°F for two days or more
- sore throat persists
- persistent cough keeps a child awake
- cough produces colored mucus for more than two days
- severe headaches, stiff neck, swollen glands, or rash are present

If anyone has a cold that doesn't seem to be getting better after five to seven days, or if there are any complications such as high fever, chest pain, or difficulty in breathing, a doctor should be called at once. Secondary infections are not common with colds, but they can occur. Bronchitis, sinusitis, tonsillitis, ear infections, and pneumonia are bacterial infections that can develop when the body is weakened by a cold, and they are often best treated when detected early.

Secondary bacterial infections *can* be treated with antibiotics. These drugs work by preventing bacteria from using energy and reproducing. But viruses reproduce only when inside other living cells. Only a few medicines are known to be able to affect viruses without also harming the cells they have infected. For most people with colds the doctor can't do much more than advise getting plenty of rest, drinking plenty of fluids, keeping warm, and taking over-the-counter medications for cold symptoms.

Coping With a Cold

Rest is important for treating a cold. Feeling tired when we're sick is a signal that we need to slow down and rest. This will help the body rebuild its strength while it fights the viruses within us. Vigorous exertion during an illness can lower the body's defenses, possibly making a cold worse. Staying home when we first feel symptoms also helps to prevent spreading cold germs.

Fluids. It was once believed that drinking lots of fluids could wash away a cold. Although this isn't true, it is

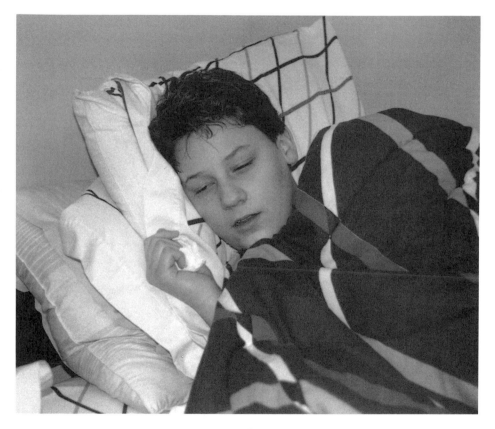

Rest is important for treating a cold.

important to drink plenty of liquids, such as water, fruit juices, tea, and broth. This will help to prevent the dehydration that may result from a fever, and it will also help to loosen sticky mucus in the breathing passageways. When the bronchial passages become blocked by thick mucus, complications such as bronchitis and pneumonia are more likely. Some doctors advise drinking eight ounces of hot liquid every two hours to meet the body's extra fluid needs, as well as to help soothe the throat and open up congested nasal passages. (Keeping the head elevated also helps to ease the congestion.)

When Grandma says to drink chicken soup for a cold, she's in good company. As far back as two thousand years ago, physicians recommended chicken soup for colds. In 1978 a study conducted by Dr. Marvin Sackner of Mount Sinai Hospital in Miami Beach, Florida, found that chicken soup really did help clear nasal mucus faster than other liquids.[6]

Many people think that you should not drink milk or eat dairy products when you have a cold because they produce more mucus. However, a study conducted at the University of Adelaide in Australia found that dairy products do not increase mucus production.[7]

Keeping warm. Being cold may not cause colds, but keeping warm (though not too hot) helps the body maintain its internal temperature with less effort, so that it is free to concentrate on more important matters—such as fighting cold viruses! John La Montagne, a virologist at the National Institutes of Health, takes a hot shower when he has a cold because hot temperatures kill rhinoviruses (at least in test tubes) and drinks a lot of water, hot soup, and juices to loosen phlegm.[8] Gargling with warm salt water or sucking on hard candies may also be effective for relieving minor sore throat pain.

Feed a cold . . . Colds can sometimes make us lose our appetites. But it's especially important to eat a nutritious diet when we have a cold. The body may need even more vitamins and minerals than normal when it is fighting off disease. Nutrition experts such as Dr. Judith Wurtman at Massachusetts Institute of Technology, advise eating easy-to-swallow foods with lots of protein, vitamins, and minerals when we're sick. Pureed meat and vegetable soups, yogurt or cottage cheese, scrambled eggs, protein drinks, baked potatoes, custard, and hot breakfast cereals are some of the foods she recommends. Vitamin and mineral supplements may also be advisable during colds, especially when we feel as if we can't eat.[9]

OTC Medications

Although many doctors feel it's best to wait out a simple cold, many people find the waiting period is just too miserable to endure without some help. Over-the-counter (OTC) medicines promise to get rid of cold symptoms quickly, and there are more than eight hundred different brands and combinations to choose from.[10] That's why Americans spend three billion dollars each year on over-the-counter medications. These drugs can help to relieve symptoms, but many doctors advise that they be used with care; remember that symptoms such as runny nose, congestion, coughing, and sneezing are part of the body's defense against colds.

Some of the most popular medications contain many different drugs to treat a whole variety of symptoms. But most colds cause only a few symptoms. "Very few patients need more than one ingredient," says Robert Couch, chairman of microbiology and immunology at Baylor College of Medicine in Houston.[11] In 1972 the Food and Drug Administration (FDA), the government agency that oversees drugs, brought together an expert panel to decide which over-the-counter cold remedies were safe and effective. The panel decided that multisymptom products were usually unnecessary. Use a decongestant nasal spray for a stuffed-up nose, or a throat lozenge for a sore throat, if recommended, rather than taking a medication that contains decongestant, antihistamine, pain reliever, and cough suppressant all in one. Drugs can produce side effects, such as drowsiness, fast heartbeat, and high blood pressure, and they are more likely with multidrug shotgun medicines. And most cold remedies don't really help very much. Dr. Gwaltney points out that over-the-counter medications "are probably safe, but they're not very effective."[12]

Some doctors think it is better not to use medications at all for the common cold, especially for children. "Using OTC medications for children can make the child's condition worse," says Florida pediatrician Dr. Angel Cadiz. "Certainly for children under six months of age, I recommend no OTC

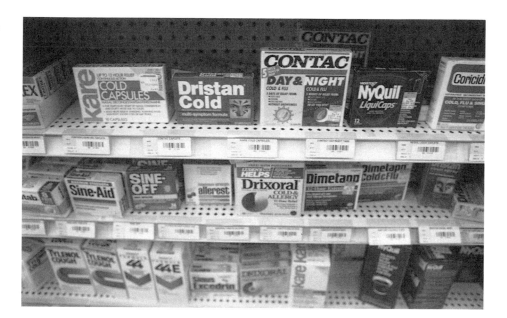

There are over 800 brands and combinations of over-the-counter medications available today. Many doctors recommend that these be used sparingly.

decongestants or antihistamines. It's really better for the illness to run its course."[13] Many experts agree. Dr. Nancy Hutton and other researchers at the Johns Hopkins Children's Center found that more than half of the children were better two days after going to the doctor, whether or not the parents had given their children any medication.[14]

Decongestants. The FDA panel found that decongestants can help clear a stuffy nose. Decongestants reduce nasal stuffiness and congestion by shrinking blood vessels in the nose. This allows mucus to drain more effectively, making it easier to breathe. But decongestant sprays should not be used more than three days in a row because they can lead to a

THE RIGHT WAY TO BLOW

Experts advise against blowing the nose too hard—it can strain blood vessels in the nose, and may even force infected mucus into the sinuses or ears, causing complications. The proper way to blow is to hold the tissue before the nostrils and exhale softly, touching raw skin under the nose as little as possible. Disposable tissues are better than handkerchiefs because cold viruses can survive for hours in a handkerchief.

condition called rebound congestion, in which the blood vessels overreact and swell up unless more decongestant is used. Some decongestants can also cause side effects such as high blood pressure, insomnia, nervousness, or reduced appetite.

Antihistamines. Scientists used to think that many cold symptoms, such as runny nose and congestion, were caused by substances in the body called histamines. Histamines produce coldlike symptoms during an allergic reaction. But more recent studies have found that bradykinins, proteins that are one hundred times more powerful than histamines, are actually responsible for cold symptoms. This explains why numerous studies over the past two decades have concluded that while antihistamines help reduce allergy symptoms, they do not relieve cold symptoms.[15] Numerous experts have warned against antihistamines, including the 1972 FDA panel, a 1988 panel of experts who met at the Children's Hospital in Pittsburgh, Pennsylvania, and scientists testifying before Congress in 1992.

However, many over-the-counter remedies still contain antihistamines. In addition to being ineffective, they can produce side effects such as drowsiness, dry mouth, nervousness, and impaired mental functioning.

Cough medicines. Two main types of cough medicines are available. Cough suppressants dull the part of the brain that causes coughing. Coughs that bring up mucus should not be treated with cough suppressants, because mucus can get thicker and plug up the air passages, making complications more likely. Cough suppressants may be helpful with a dry cough, though, especially when it interferes with sleep. Expectorants loosen mucus so that it can be coughed up more easily, but several studies and the 1972 FDA panel did not find that expectorants helped relieve common cold symptoms.

Some Controversial Remedies

Humidifier. Some doctors believe that humidifiers can help relieve congestion and throat pain, by moistening the nasal and throat tissues. But others say that humidifiers have the potential to cause more harm than good. Bacteria and fungi can multiply in moist humidifiers, and then be inhaled along with the steam or mist. Unless humidifiers are cleaned thoroughly and often, they can cause allergic reactions or secondary infections.

Hot air. Some researchers have found that raising the temperature of the nasal lining (local hyperthermia) may be helpful in treating colds. In a 1987 study conducted by Israeli researchers, for example, cold sufferers inhaled moist hot air for two 20-minute sessions after a cold had started and found their nasal symptoms improved, even for several days afterwards.[16] A popular device for self-administering hot, moist air was claimed to greatly shorten the duration of colds and relieve stuffiness. However, other studies, such as one conducted by researchers at the Cleveland Clinic in Ohio, found no beneficial effects from inhaling moist, hot air. In fact, they found that hot, humid air may even damage the nasal tissue.[17]

Zinc. In a clinical trial at the University of Texas in 1984, sucking on zinc gluconate tablets helped cold sufferers get over colds more quickly. Zinc is an essential mineral, involved in many important enzyme reactions in the body and in the work of the immune system. But too much of it can produce serious side effects, such as a general sick feeling, nausea, vomiting, and blood-cell damage. By the early 1990s many doctors had dismissed zinc lozenges as a possible remedy for colds. But in 1992 Dr. Nancy Jane Godfrey published a study conducted among students at Dartmouth College that found sucking on zinc gluconate lozenges at the first sign of colds halved the amount of time that students were sick.[18]

Herbs. Herbs have been used to treat cold symptoms for thousands of years by many different cultures. Many herbal remedies are still used today. Various teas, for example, are said to help cold symptoms. These may contain substances such as peppermint oil (which contains menthol to help ease coughing), the Chinese herb mahuang (which contains ephedra, a natural decongestant), and slippery elm, which soothes sore throats. One of the most popular is echinacea, or purple coneflower, which has been used by Native Americans for centuries for everything from snakebites to infections and burns. This herb was an ingredient in many of the cure-alls of the 1800s and until the 1920s it was the most widely used herbal remedy in America. Today, this native American herb is very popular in Europe, particularly in Germany, where it can be found in hundreds of medicines. Scientific studies conducted by

German scientists over the past fifty years suggest that echinacea may have antibiotic, antiviral, wound-healing, and anti-inflammatory powers, and may be useful as an immune booster to help prevent colds and the flu.[19] However, this herb remains almost untested by the American scientific community.

6

Preventing Colds

We live in a world filled with colds just waiting to happen. For most people colds are not serious illnesses. But for some, such as those with chronic heart or lung disease, any infection—even "just a cold"—can be dangerous. For such people, avoiding colds can be a life-and-death matter.

How Can We Prevent Colds?

The only sure way to avoid catching a cold is to stay away from anyone who has one, or any place they have recently visited. But there are things you can do to prevent colds without isolating yourself from the world. They fall into two categories: (1) reducing opportunities for colds to spread, and (2) keeping yourself healthy so that you can fight off cold germs if you do become infected.

To stop cold viruses from spreading to you, you can avoid contact with people who have colds, wash your hands regularly, and avoid touching your eyes or nose before washing your hands. Washing your hands won't kill cold viruses, but it *will* wash them down the drain. If you are the one with a cold, washing your hands often can help to avoid sharing your viruses with others. (Remember that cold viruses are spread both by air and hand-to-hand.) When family members have colds, it may be a good idea for the sick person to have his or her own towel until the cold is over.

Keeping yourself healthy will also help protect against colds by keeping your resistance up. You promote good health by eating sensibly, exercising regularly, getting enough rest, and practicing cleanliness (washing hands and keeping body, clothes, food, and dishes clean).

In a recent study at the University of California School of Medicine at Davis, Dr. Georges Halpern tested a folk remedy, yogurt, on 120 volunteers of various ages, from young adult to elderly. Those who ate six ounces of yogurt every day for a year had 25 percent fewer colds than those who did not. The researcher has found that the live microbes in yogurt stimulate the production of gamma interferon, one of the body's immune defenses.[1]

Helping to reduce stress can also boost the immune system. Dr. R. C. Green of Harvard University found that after volunteers relaxed for twenty minutes with their eyes closed, stress was reduced and body levels of immunoglobulin increased.[2]

Benjamin Franklin believed that fresh air prevents colds. He was right. Fresh air helps to dilute virus particles in the air and make it less likely for them to be inhaled. One study revealed another way that fresh air can help prevent colds and other respiratory diseases. At the University of California at Berkeley, Dr. Albert P. Krueger found that air molecules called ions have a negative electrical charge in fresh air, but are positively charged when in smoky, stale air. In his experiments a machine that produces negative ions was found to help prevent colds. Dr. Krueger believes that negative ions may increase the body's levels of serotonin, a chemical that is important for the immune system.[3]

THE PROS AND CONS OF BEING POLITE

Covering the mouth when coughing or sneezing started out as a superstition, but today it is a part of polite behavior. If you sneeze into the air, the droplets will settle to the ground, but sneezing into your hand concentrates germs that might then be picked up by someone else. So should you cover or not cover? The best answer: Cover your mouth and then wash your hands!

It's also polite behavior to shake hands with people, but many experts advise that it's "cold-smart" to greet people with words alone during the cold season.

Some experts recommend taking vitamin supplements to keep the immune system strong. But others advise against vitamin supplements, stating that a proper diet provides all the nutrients we need to be healthy.

Vitamin C. In 1970, Linus Pauling, a Nobel Prize-wining chemist at Stanford University, published a book called *Vitamin C and the Common Cold,* in which he claimed that large doses of vitamin C (150 times the dose the government recommends for daily nutrition) could raise our resistance and prevent or reduce the severity of a cold. According to Pauling, by strengthening the protein "glue" the holds body cells together, vitamin C hinders the movement of viruses through tissues and into cells. This vitamin also strengthens the body's immune defenses and may be linked to interferon formation and activity.[4]

Pauling's book generated a huge controversy among doctors and scientists. Some said the "megadoses" that Pauling recommends could not have a protective effect because the body rids itself of excess vitamin C, producing what one researcher called "very expensive urine."[5] And such large doses of the vitamin could produce unpleasant or even dangerous side effects, including diarrhea, kidney stones, and blood-clotting problems. People who take high levels of vitamin C supplements may become dependent on them and then suffer from scurvy, a vitamin C deficiency disease, if they go back to the "normal" dietary amounts.[6]

Experiments were conducted to determine whether vitamin C really does help to prevent colds. Some seemed to support Linus Pauling's view but others did not. One major study was sponsored in the 1980s by Hoffmann-LaRoche. Dr. Elliot Dick of the respiratory virus research laboratory at the University of Wisconsin gave volunteers two grams of vitamin C for three weeks, then placed the subjects in a weekend-long poker game with infected volunteers. Although the vitamin C users became infected, Dr. Dick points out that "their symptoms were much, much milder."[7] "They had fewer coughs, and they didn't blow their noses as often, which are objective measures of severity," says Dr. Dick.[8] The researcher was skeptical before the trial, but now he takes vitamin C to protect himself against colds.[9]

Interferon. Since 1957 some scientists have believed that interferon, a natural immune-boosting substance produced in the body, might be the ultimate cure for the common cold. But interferon could only be extracted from white blood cells and was very expensive to make in the laboratory. (In a 1973 study, tests of interferon cost $3,000 per person!) So studies of this cold preventative were abandoned until the late 1970s, when genetic engineering made it possible to produce interferons more cheaply. In studies published in 1986, synthetic interferon, given in a nasal spray, helped reduce the spread of colds among family members by 40 percent. But it was still quite expensive—it cost nearly $250 to prevent each cold in this study. There were also unpleasant side effects, and interferon was effective only against rhinoviruses. So the makers of the drug dropped the cold studies and focused their efforts on interferon's effects against other viruses.[10]

Dr. Gwaltney of the University of Virginia has tested a "cocktail" that combines interferon with two anti-inflammatory drugs. Patients were given the combination drug after cold symptoms had started. The drug mixture acts to stop both the cause (the virus) and the effect (inflammation). The interferon reduced viral shedding, and the anti-inflammatory drugs helped the patients to feel better.[11]

Don't Put a Cold in Your Pocket

When handkerchiefs were invented a few centuries ago, they were a big improvement in public health. (Until then, people wiped runny noses on their sleeves.) But hankies have some disadvantages. Each time you use one, it gets a little more contaminated with cold viruses, and every time you reach into your pocket for it your hands get more gooey. Besides, University of Virginia researchers have found that viruses survive for quite a while on cloth hankies. Paper tissues, on the other hand, absorb viruses better and seem to neutralize them within a few hours.[12] Paper tissues are disposable and you throw them away after you use them, so there are fewer chances of passing viruses to other people.

At the University of Wisconsin, Dr. Elliot Dick came up with an even better tissue. He has tested tissues treated with citric and malic acid (both are natural chemicals found in fruits) and a mild detergent called sodium lauryl sulfate. The treated tissues killed 100 percent of rhinoviruses and 80 percent of other cold viruses that were blown into them. When volunteers with colds played poker with healthy

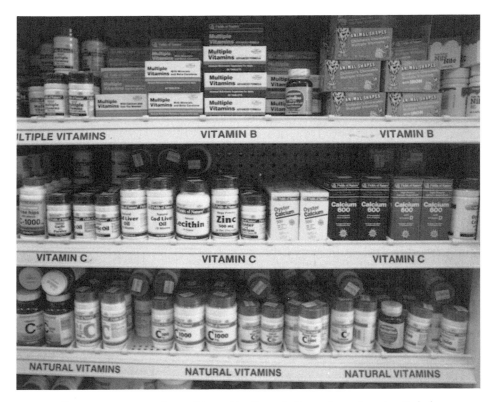

Some experts, such as Linus Pauling, believe that vitamin C helps prevent colds.

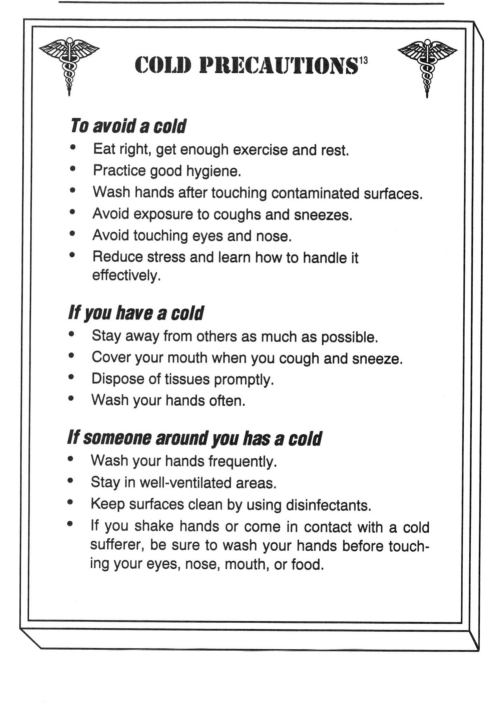

COLD PRECAUTIONS[13]

To avoid a cold

- Eat right, get enough exercise and rest.
- Practice good hygiene.
- Wash hands after touching contaminated surfaces.
- Avoid exposure to coughs and sneezes.
- Avoid touching eyes and nose.
- Reduce stress and learn how to handle it effectively.

If you have a cold

- Stay away from others as much as possible.
- Cover your mouth when you cough and sneeze.
- Dispose of tissues promptly.
- Wash your hands often.

If someone around you has a cold

- Wash your hands frequently.
- Stay in well-ventilated areas.
- Keep surfaces clean by using disinfectants.
- If you shake hands or come in contact with a cold sufferer, be sure to wash your hands before touching your eyes, nose, mouth, or food.

volunteers and used the tissues every time they sneezed or blew their noses, none of the healthy volunteers caught colds. When cold-infected volunteers used handkerchiefs instead, 42 to 75 percent of the healthy volunteers caught colds.

Kimberly Clark test-marketed the tissues in 1984, but consumer did not want to pay two to three times the price of regular tissues, and the product was dropped.[14] Some experts believe that the tissues were dropped too quickly and hope they will eventually be reintroduced.

Other researchers are testing antiviral soaps that kill viruses on the hands, and Dr. Dick is testing to see whether an air filter will help suck viruses out of the air to prevent the transmission of colds.

Knowledge Is Power

Although there is not yet a cure for the common cold, nor a vaccine to prevent it, knowing what to do can help make colds less severe and prevent serious complications. A study reported in the *Journal of the American Medical Association* in 1983 found that when health clinics gave information about colds to their patients, there were 40 percent fewer visits to the doctor for cold symptoms. The informed patients spent less money on cold medicines, too, and were less worried about their colds.[15]

THE FLU

What is it? An infectious disease caused by influenza A or B virus; highly contagious and tends to spread in epidemics; affects the upper respiratory tract; may spread to the lungs.

Who gets it? All ages, all races, both sexes; most dangerous to the elderly, those with chronic diseases, and the immune-suppressed, who may develop more serious secondary complications.

How do you get it? Mainly by breathing virus-contaminated droplets; also spread by hand contact.

What are the symptoms? Headaches, chills, muscle aches, cough, sore throat, and fever; congestion may also be present. Illness usually begins suddenly. Body temperature returns to normal by the fourth day; other symptoms may persist for a week. Diarrhea, nausea, and vomiting are rare in adults. ("Stomach flu" is usually some other infection.)

How is it treated? Rest, drinking plenty of fluids, and over-the-counter medications for symptoms. Those at high risk for complications may be treated with antiviral medications such as amantadine and rimantadine. Complications are treated with antibiotics.

How can it be prevented? Flu vaccines are available to protect against the virus strains currently in circulation. (Protective antibodies take about two weeks to build up.) Vaccination is highly recommended for those most at risk for complications.

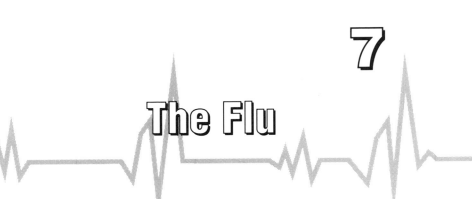

The Flu

I t started in an army camp at Fort Riley, Kansas, in March of 1918. Some soldiers began complaining of chills and fever, aching head and muscles, and sore throats. By the end of the week, more than five hundred men at the fort were sick, and soon a dozen other overcrowded military camps were also struck. At Fort Riley forty-six men died of pneumonia complications, but the Army didn't pay much attention. There was a war going on. Men were shipped overseas in crowded conditions.

By that fall, the servicemen had carried the flu to France—but now it was much worse. Symptoms included dizziness, vomiting, sweating, and difficulty in breathing. Large numbers of people began to die, often quite quickly and with extensive lung damage. The second wave spread from France to England and then to Spain, where it killed eight million Spaniards and acquired the popular name of "Spanish flu." The disease spread eastward to the German army in Germany, then to Russia, China, Japan, and down to South Africa, across to India, and then to South America.

Back in the United States, the flu was at first confined to the Army, but in early September 1918 the first civilian case was reported in Boston. The disease spread quickly. By the end of September ten thousand Americans had died. Poor sanitary conditions and the scarcity of doctors and nurses (many of whom were needed in the war effort) helped the epidemic to spread speedily. By the end of 1918, three hundred thousand Americans had died. A third wave of flu swept the world after the end of the war and ended abruptly in the spring of 1919. By then the U.S. death toll had reached half a million.

History's Second Worst Disease

Whether you call it "a bug," "the flu," or "la grippe," influenza is a common illness that causes a lot of misery. The killer epidemic that swept through the world in the winter of 1918–19 was the second worst outbreak of any infectious disease in recorded history. In fact, it was classified as a pandemic—an infectious disease that spreads all around the world, involving millions of people. (The prefix *pan-* means "everywhere.")

Only the Black Death, the outbreak of bubonic plague that devastated fourteenth-century Europe, killed more people than the "Spanish flu." Twenty percent of all the people in the world who were alive at the time had the flu during that postwar

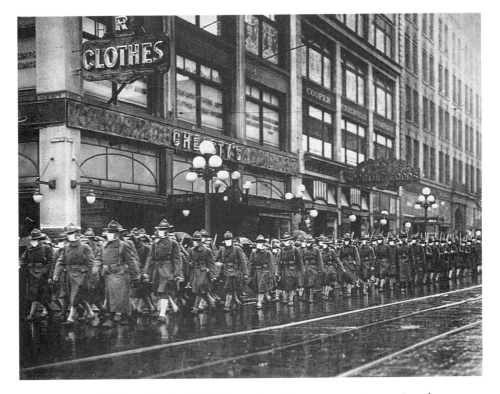

During the flu epidemic of 1918, people took extra precautions against the disease. Here, soldiers from the 39th Field Artillery Regiment are seen wearing gauze masks to prevent them from breathing contaminated air.

PICTURES FROM AN EPIDEMIC

During the influenza epidemic of 1918–19, panicked officials tried to stop the spread of disease. People were fined for spitting in public or for sneezing or coughing without a handkerchief. Health officials advised that everyone should get plenty of rest, eat regularly, and "beware of persons shaking hands."[1] The New York Commissioner of Health suggested that "any fellow kissing a girl would be wise to do it through a handkerchief."[2]

Phone booths were boarded up, and dance halls, pool rooms, movie houses, libraries, ice cream parlors, churches, and saloons were closed. In Prescott, Arizona, a person who shook hands could be thrown in jail. At a West Coast naval base, drinking fountains were blowtorched every hour to sanitize them, phones were cleaned with alcohol, and guards were ordered to shoot to kill anyone who came or went without permission.

In many places people were required to wear gauze face masks. In some cities no one could get on a bus or trolley without wearing one. In Tucson a judge fined a window washer for taking off his mask to blow a windowpane dry. San Francisco police complained that robbers were taking advantage of the masks to commit more crimes.[3]

winter! At least 20 million people died from complications developing from this worldwide outbreak—more than twice as many as were killed in World War I.

Why Influenza Can Kill

Like the common cold, the influenza virus affects the membrane cells of the nose and throat. Both illnesses destroy epithelial (lining) cells and the cilia that move mucus along. But symptoms are much worse with the flu. Unlike a cold, fever is often the first sign of influenza. (Fever may reach 104°F.)

Most people are very ill for two to four days and recover in one to two weeks without any lasting effects, but about one percent of flu sufferers develop complications. The influenza virus may spread into the lungs, causing pneumonia. If this happens it usually does so quickly—a day to a day and a half after symptoms begin—and it can be so overwhelming that it leads to death in the aged or people in poor health.

Bacterial infections, such as ear infections, sinusitis, bronchitis, and pneumonia are more common with the flu than with colds, and may develop three or four days after the influenza begins. Instead of getting better, the person gets sicker. Doctors have also discovered that heart failure and other chronic diseases are an even greater cause of flu-related deaths than pneumonia. The stress on the body of a person with heart problems or other chronic ailments can often prove too great. Each year an average of twenty thousand Americans die (fifty thousand in an epidemic year), not necessarily from the flu but from flu complications.[4]

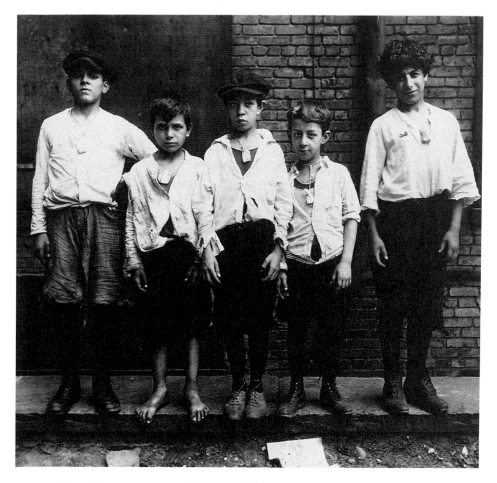

These boys wore camphor around their necks during the 1918 flu epidemic, hoping it would prevent them from catching the flu.

Usually the flu is most dangerous for the very young and the very old. From 75 to 90 percent of influenza-related deaths occur in people sixty-five or over.[5] But the Spanish flu was different. This strain was deadly for those in the prime of life. In San Francisco, for example, two-thirds of the people who died were between twenty and forty. Similar statistics were found in other cities.

The Flu Viruses

Until 1918, scientists thought that influenza was caused by bacteria, but no bacterial infection was found in autopsies. During the 1918 pandemic, J. S. Koen, a veterinarian of the U.S. Bureau of Animal Industry in Iowa, noticed that a disease in pigs resembled the Spanish flu. He noted that in places where pigs and people lived close together, an outbreak in the family would be followed by an outbreak among the pigs, or vice versa. His observation was largely ignored until 1931, when Richard Shope, a pathologist at the Rockefeller Institute for Comparative Pathology in Princeton, New Jersey, passed mucus from sick pigs through a filter and then placed it in the noses of healthy pigs, which then became ill, thus proving that swine flu was spread by a virus.

In 1933 British researchers Wilson Smith and Christopher Andrewes discovered the first human flu virus. Andrewes had a case of the flu, so Smith placed drops of his throat washings in the noses of ferrets. The animals were soon suffering from fever, sneezing, and runny noses, just like human flu victims. Studies of the disease continued, and several years later the flu virus was successfully grown in chicken eggs.

Researchers ultimately discovered that there are three different types of viruses that can cause flu in humans. The one that the British team worked on was named influenza A. During the 1940s, influenza B and then influenza C were discovered. Influenza viruses make up a family called orthomyxoviruses, and they are slightly larger than cold viruses.

Influenza B and C are usually found only in humans. Influenza A is the most dangerous and is found in many animals such as birds, horses, seals, swine, and whales.

Influenza A is the type that causes pandemics. Influenza A

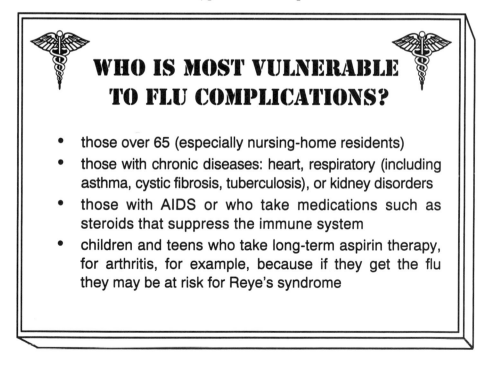

WHO IS MOST VULNERABLE TO FLU COMPLICATIONS?

- those over 65 (especially nursing-home residents)
- those with chronic diseases: heart, respiratory (including asthma, cystic fibrosis, tuberculosis), or kidney disorders
- those with AIDS or who take medications such as steroids that suppress the immune system
- children and teens who take long-term aspirin therapy, for arthritis, for example, because if they get the flu they may be at risk for Reye's syndrome

and B produce very similar symptoms, but influenza B causes less severe epidemics and rarely affects adults. Influenza B has also been associated with Reye's syndrome, which may occur in one out of every twenty thousand cases of influenza B in children. Influenza C rarely causes disease.

What Does the Flu Virus Look Like?

The flu virus is covered with a fatty envelope with two types of protein molecules sticking out in hundreds of spikes. One type of spike is called a hemagglutinin molecule (H spike) because it combines with red blood cells and causes them to clump together. The H spike matches with proteins on the surface of respiratory cells, allowing the virus to attach itself to them. N spikes or neuraminidase molecules help the virus to get into the cells and also help in releasing virus copies from infected cells.

Inside the protective coat of a flu virus there are eight pieces of genetic material. This is very unusual for viruses. (In most viruses, the genetic material is contained in one strand.) Because the flu virus genes are divided among separate nucleic acid strands, there is a good chance that they will not line up in the right order when the virus reproduces. As a result, the new viruses may not be exact copies of the original. Hence, flu viruses mutate (change) more than other kinds of viruses, producing changes in the spikes in the virus's outer coat.

The human immune system recognizes a flu virus by its spikes and makes antibodies to match up to the amino acids

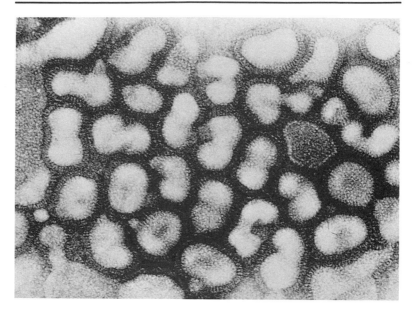

The Influenza A virus, greatly magnified. This was the first of the influenza viruses to be discovered by researchers in the 1930s.

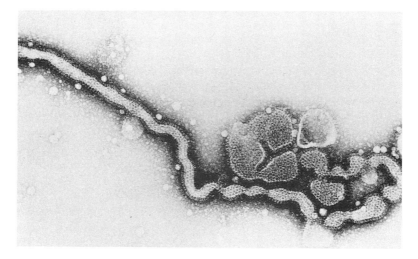

The Influenza C virus, greatly magnified. This strain of the virus rarely causes disease.

that make up the spike proteins. The greater the changes in the flu virus spikes, the less likely it is that the body will be able to use antibodies it has built up from previous infections to stop the new viruses. That is why immunity to influenza is generally not as long-lasting as immunity to other diseases.

About one percent of the amino acids on the spikes of flu viruses mutate each year. This gradual change is called antigenic drift; eventually the small changes can build up to make the virus quite different. Even these small changes can be enough to produce new flu outbreaks every year. But flu viruses can also mutate abruptly, producing a completely new hemagglutinin, neuraminidase, or both. Such a sudden, dramatic change is called antigenic shift. When it occurs, the whole world is exposed to an influenza A virus with H or N spikes that have never been encountered before, so no one has antibody protection, and a flu outbreak can rapidly develop into a sweeping epidemic. Antigenic shifts occurred in 1918, 1957, and 1968. Strangely, the old influenza A virus disappeared each time, and only the new one remained in circulation.

Scientists used to think that shifts were just the result of many drifts, but researchers have found this is not the case. When an antigenic shift occurs, the new strain is very different from the old one. In 1968 when a new flu strain arose, 70 percent of the amino acids in the new H spike were different from the strain that was in circulation the year before![6]

81

In 1957 45 million Americans came down with the Asian flu, and seventy thousand people died.[7] The next antigenic shift, in 1968, resulted in the Hong Kong flu, which struck one-quarter of all Americans but killed only about thirty-four thousand.[8] Why was the Hong Kong flu epidemic less severe? Researchers think the reason was that although the H spike had changed, the N spike stayed the same as in the Asian flu, so people had at least some protection.

The flu doesn't kill people just during worldwide pandemics. The same virus that caused the 1968 pandemic killed three hundred thousand Americans between 1968 and 1990, when no major pandemics were occurring. This strain is the deadliest flu virus around today.

In 1977 influenza researchers were surprised to discover that the influenza A virus that had been around in the early 1950s had reemerged, but the current A strain did not disappear. These two influenza A strains and an influenza B strain are currently circulating.

Keeping an Eye on the Flu

The World Health Organization (WHO) has been monitoring influenza viruses since 1947. More than two hundred influenza centers worldwide send virus samples to WHO centers in London, Melbourne, Australia, or Atlanta, Georgia. Viruses are tested there and each is given a name, which includes the virus type and the place it is from. This is how virus strains come to be known by popular names such as Hong Kong flu, Shanghai flu, etc.

When the WHO finds different variations of circulating strains, they are stored at extremely low temperatures for future use. Scientists hope to use these samples to understand how the influenza virus evolves.

Where Do New Flu Strains Come From?

Scientists believe that new influenza strains develop when an animal or human is infected with two different flu viruses—one that affects only humans and one that affects only animals. The two strains crossbreed or reshuffle, producing new hybrid viruses that are able to infect humans.

Another theory is that a flu virus becomes so common in humans that it can no longer cause infection because everyone has built up antibodies. So it then infects animals such as ducks or pigs. After a few generations, most people no longer have antibodies against that particular virus, and it returns to attack humans again. This is the "barnyard storage" theory.

The 1957 and 1968 influenza pandemics were traced to China, and the 1977 Russian flu is also believed to have originated in China. One reason may be that the crossbreeding of animal and human viruses or barnyard storage is more likely to occur in a country like China, where many people live in close contact with domesticated animals such as pigs and ducks.

When Does the Flu Occur?

Flu epidemics generally occur in the winter months. From 10 to 40 percent of the U.S. population is affected each year over a period of six to twelve weeks.[9] In the Northern Hemisphere the flu season is normally from December to April, except during pandemics, when the disease spreads from early autumn to late spring.

The flu spreads best in cold weather because people are crowded indoors more often, giving the virus a better chance to spread. Also the lower humidity in wintertime dries out nasal mucous membranes, and viruses can get past the defenses more easily.

How Is the Flu Spread?

Influenza is spread through aerosolized droplets that are produced when an infected person coughs, sneezes, or even talks. Flu viruses travel better through the air than cold viruses do. Cold germs can only float on fairly large droplets after a sneeze or a cough, but flu viruses can also travel on very small droplets, which are able to remain in the air for much longer periods of time. Like colds, the flu is also spread by hand contact.

The flu can spread quickly in closed-in spaces such as classrooms, offices, buses, stores, restaurants, and theaters. In 1979, for example, a passenger with the flu boarded an airplane for a five-hour flight. Within three days, 72 percent of the other fifty-three passengers on the plane came down with the flu.[10] Infected people can spread the virus before they have symptoms—or without even having symptoms. Many may have mild symptoms and think they only have a slight cold.

Seeing a Doctor

A doctor should be consulted:

- if flu symptoms last more than a week;

- if symptoms becomes severe or localized in the throat, stomach, or lungs:

- if other symptoms such as a fever of 103°F or more develop;

- if fever returns after symptoms seem to have been getting better;

- if vomiting and behavioral changes occur; or

- if someone at high risk for complications gets the flu.

Diagnosing the Flu

Doctors can diagnose influenza with laboratory tests, but these were rarely done until recently. Influenza tests were expensive and results took up to a week to obtain; by then the illness was mostly over. Doctors usually made a clinical diagnosis, based on symptoms and whether or not influenza was occurring in the area.

In 1990 a new test, which gives doctors results in 15 minutes, was approved by the FDA. Manufactured by Beckton Dickinson, the test costs less than $20. The nose is rinsed with a salt solution, and then the solution is tested for flu virus. This faster test is being used more often now to confirm the flu. However, the test only identifies influenza type A viruses, not influenza B or common cold viruses.[11]

Treatment for the Flu

Flu complications such as ear infections, sinusitis, bronchitis, and pneumonia may be treated with antibiotics. But if these complications are not present, for many patients the doctor may prescribe the same treatment for the flu as for a cold: plenty of rest, plenty of fluids, and over-the-counter medications.

Antiviral drugs. For those at risk for complications the doctor may prescribe a drug called amantadine. This drug seems to keep influenza A viruses from reproducing, but it is not effective with influenza B viruses. If taken within the first day or two after symptoms begin, it can reduce the severity of the illness and get it over with more quickly.

Amantadine can be 70 to 90 percent effective in preventing type A influenza from developing, but it has to be taken every day for the entire flu season. Rimantadine has also been approved for flu prevention and treatment. Some researchers are worried that resistance to these antiviral drugs may develop. Influenza A viruses that are resistant to these drugs have been found in patients taking them, but researchers are not sure how much of a threat in terms of spreading these drug-resistant viruses constitute.

Keep warm but not too warm. It's important to keep warm when you have the flu, but turning up the heat too high when you're sick may not be a good idea. Dr. David Fairbanks, spokesperson for the American Academy of Otolaryngology—Head and Neck Surgery points out that cool air helps shrink blood vessels in the nose, which helps you to breathe more easily. The head and feet should be kept warm, however.[12]

What about exercise? For most people who have the flu and are suffering from muscle aches and extreme fatigue, vigorous exercise is the last thing on their minds. But some people who regularly exercise vigorously may feel driven to get back into their normal routine as quickly as possible. Some studies have found that moderate exercise when the patient feels up to it is not harmful. But according to a study done in Nova Scotia, one out of ten flu sufferers may suffer temporary inflammation of the heart, due to the fever the illness brings with it. Dr. Thomas Marrie at Dalhousie University Faculty of Medicine in Halifax

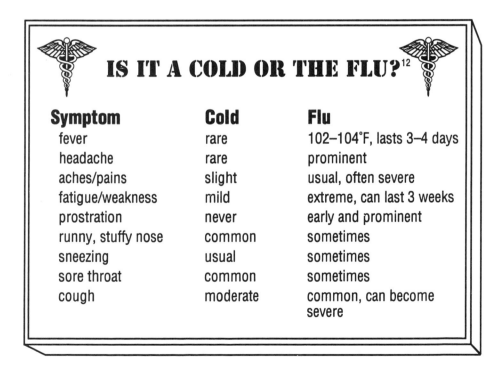

IS IT A COLD OR THE FLU?[12]

Symptom	Cold	Flu
fever	rare	102–104°F, lasts 3–4 days
headache	rare	prominent
aches/pains	slight	usual, often severe
fatigue/weakness	mild	extreme, can last 3 weeks
prostration	never	early and prominent
runny, stuffy nose	common	sometimes
sneezing	usual	sometimes
sore throat	common	sometimes
cough	moderate	common, can become severe

warns, "If you're used to running five or six miles a day, don't do it for at least two weeks, possibly four, after the symptoms clear."[14]

Preventing the Flu

For many, the flu can be a serious illness, and each year millions of people receive flu vaccinations. Flu vaccines are made up of "killed" or inactivated virus. People have to get a new flu vaccine each year because flu viruses change each season. (For other viral infections, such as German measles and polio, a single vaccination is good for a lifetime.)

Each winter experts from the FDA, CDC, the WHO, and other medical groups plan the new year's vaccine. They look at the viruses currently circulating in the Northern Hemisphere and those from the previous season in the Southern Hemisphere, because its flu season usually has not started when the decision must be made. The current influenza viruses are combined with older ones, using genetic technology, and grown in fertilized chicken eggs. Then the viruses are inactivated or killed so that they cannot reproduce but will still stimulate antibody production. Recent vaccines contain killed versions of three different viruses. When the prediction is accurate, up to 70 percent of those inoculated will not get the flu.

Because the vaccine is chosen months in advance, sometimes the virus changes before the flu season starts, and the vaccine will not be effective. However, even if this happens, the vaccine usually makes the illness less severe and reduces the likelihood of developing complications. In elderly and immune-suppressed

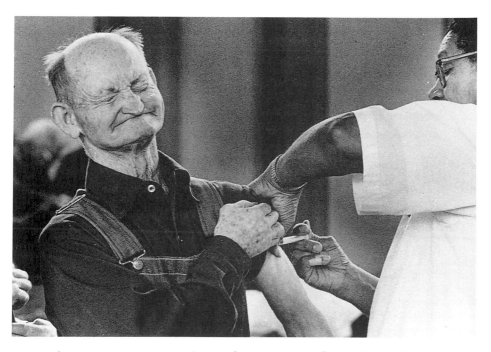

Flu vaccinations are a good way of preventing the flu. Adults usually get one flu shot per year.

people, vaccines are more effective in preventing death-causing complications than in preventing the flu itself.

The first effective flu vaccine was produced in 1944 and was used on American troops during World War II. In spite of the wartime conditions, there was no major flu outbreak.

Adults usually get one flu shot; children under nine get two if they are receiving an influenza vaccination for the first time. Two weeks after the shot, antibodies are usually present in the person's bloodstream; they provide protection for about six months and then become less effective. However, many people who ought to be vaccinated don't bother to get shots. According to the CDC, only 30 percent of those at greatest risk for complications are vaccinated.

Perhaps the most common reason people don't get vaccinated is that they are afraid of side effects. In the past, flu vaccines were not as purified as they are now. Some people experience flulike symptoms after a shot, such as fever, muscle aches, and headaches. These people were not infected with the disease, but the vaccine contained substances that activated some of the immune responses that trigger influenza symptoms. Today most people have no side effects.

Only 1 percent of the public is advised not to get vaccines: those with severe egg allergies (most flu vaccines are grown in eggs); those who previously had an allergic reaction to a flu vaccine; and babies less than six months old.

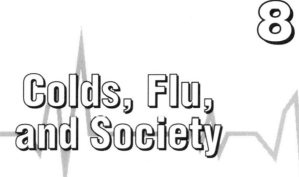

Colds, Flu, and Society

Doctors advise getting plenty of rest when you have a cold. It's a good idea—taking it easy for a few days while fighting a cold can help to strengthen your immune defenses and it also avoids spreading a highly contagious illness to other people. But how many people actually do stay in bed (or even at home) for a few days for "just a cold"? In our modern world, people have responsibilities.

If a student misses a few days of school, there will be homework to make up, and classwork will be missed completely. Or perhaps a big test is scheduled. You might not do as well as you would if you were feeling well—but you might get a zero if you don't take the test at all.

People who work have their own problems. Many people feel that it is their duty to get the job done, whether they feel well or not. Others may worry about losing pay or even getting fired if they take sick days off.

Recent Ann Landers columns have discussed the question of what is the responsible thing to do when you're sick. One letter writer pointed out that people who come in to work sick may not be able to do their jobs effectively, and they put others in danger of getting sick, too. But another reader objected, "Why doesn't she discuss this with some real-life employers? . . . Employers don't care if you are sick, they just want you to be there. Most of the time if you give in to what ails you in the early stages and take a few days off to be lazy at home, you may not end up using as many sick days as you would if you postponed the process. Your employer, however, would prefer that you gamble, and with luck you can heal on the job. You might not be quite as sharp, but you'd be there."[1]

Are We Spending Too Much Time Studying the Cold?

Some people think scientists are spending too much time trying to find a cure for the common cold. "We're dealing with a disease that is more of a nuisance than a disability. I don't see it as very high on the priority list like AIDS or some of the other viruses that are devastating," says Dr. Robert Taylor of Mary Black Memorial Hospital in Spartanburg, South Carolina.[2]

However, others see importance in cold research. "Searching for a cure for the common cold does serve a purpose in the long run. If we learn something about a given virus, then there is certainly other virus research that can benefit from that knowledge. Also, a cure for the common cold would alleviate the tremendous cost the illness generates in lost productivity and through the purchase of OTC medications," says Dr. R. Wesley Dean of St. Mary's Medical Center in Knoxville, Tennessee.[3]

A cold cure could bring huge savings to society. According to one estimate, Americans spend five billion dollars a year on doctors and medicines to treat colds; a poll conducted among office workers found that most people spend about ten dollars to fight each cold[4]—and, in all, Americans suffer about a billion colds each year. The costs of lost work time are even greater. Economists estimate that lost productivity due to colds costs U.S. businesses twelve billion dollars each year.[5]

Keeping Ahead of a Killer

Influenza causes the same kinds of costs to society as the common cold but, in addition, brings the threat of death to some of its sufferers. So the enormous efforts to fight flu epidemics are certainly worthwhile.

These efforts pay off. In 1957, for example, a new strain of influenza A appeared and spread across the world, becoming the most severe pandemic since the Spanish flu of 1918. But far fewer people died from this outbreak. One reason was that scientists around the world were able to keep ahead of the killer virus.

About thirty laboratories helped identify and trace the

outbreaks of the new strain around the world. The information was sent to the World Health Organization centers, and the spread of the disease was mapped out.

Early detection had helped the medical community gear up for the pandemic. By October 1, ten million doses of vaccine had been readied for physicians, and extra antibiotics were produced to battle complications. For the first time in medical history, the medical community was able to keep ahead of an impending influenza epidemic. Health officials were following the disease so closely that when it struck New York City in August, scientists were able to pinpoint the first carriers: eight foreign students who had arrived by plane.[6]

Since then, public health agencies around the world have continued to stay on top of the flu situation. In spite of the new strains that have appeared, some of them potentially quite deadly, the world has never again had to suffer a devastating pandemic like the one of 1918–19.

The Epidemic That Wasn't

In 1976 scientists believed that a pandemic like the one in 1918 was about to happen. At Fort Dix, New Jersey, several soldiers came down with swine flu, the virus that is believed to have caused the Spanish flu. One soldier died, and health officials warned President Gerald Ford that the disease could spread. President Ford declared, "We cannot afford to take a chance with the health of our nation."[7] A national program was begun to vaccinate everyone.

After forty-six million people (about 20 percent of the

population) had been vaccinated, however, the program was abandoned. The swine flu wasn't spreading as expected, after all. In addition, five hundred people became paralyzed as a result of a rare side effect of the vaccine, and twenty-seven of them died. (This side effect has not occurred with vaccinations since then.)

Did officials do the right thing by urging everyone to be vaccinated in 1976? Although the families of the vaccine victims might not agree, it probably was the best decision for society. If the swine flu had spread, many millions would have been protected. Even today, scientists are never exactly sure whether or not a new flu strain will spread, but each year vaccinations help millions avoid the life-threatening complications of the flu.

9

Colds, Flu, and the Future

W e know more about common cold viruses than just about any other," says Elliot Dick. "We know their shape, and we know their structure down to the atom."[1] That's why cold researchers have learned the cold is tough to beat.

Medicine has brought us a "cure" for many diseases. If you get strep throat, for example, antibiotics will help kill the bacteria that cause this disease. But curing the common cold is a different story. By the time you feel any symptoms, the body is well on its way to defeating the cold viruses. "A cure for the common cold isn't realistic because by the time you've got a cold it's too late to stop the infection. But preventing colds is another matter. There's real hope now that this will happen," says Merck Sharpe & Dohme researcher Richard Colonno.[2]

Computer-aided drug design is making it easier to find drugs to combat many diseases, including the common cold and the flu. Supercomputers that contain the most up-to-date information on molecular biology and theoretical chemistry are utilized. Detailed models of a virus are displayed on the computer screen, and drugs can be tested out on the computer before being selected for testing in the lab. This greatly speeds up the testing process.

Stopping Cold Viruses

Scientists are working on three different ways to stop cold viruses. The first is to prevent viruses from releasing their genetic material once they get inside cells. The other two involve the cellular receptor that allows viruses to enter cells in the first place. Viruses can be prevented from attaching to cell receptors by blocking either the receptor or the site on the virus that attaches to the cell receptor.

Inactivating Viruses

Michael Rossmann and his colleague Tom Smith at Purdue University, working in collaboration with the Sterling-Winthrop drug company in Rensselaer, New York, have been experimenting with drugs called capsid binders that prevent viruses from shedding their protein coats (capsids) once they are inside a cell. The drugs sink into the canyons on the surface of the virus, which contain chemical structures that are recognized by receptors on body cells. The Purdue researchers have discovered that the drugs pass through a pore into a cavity beneath the

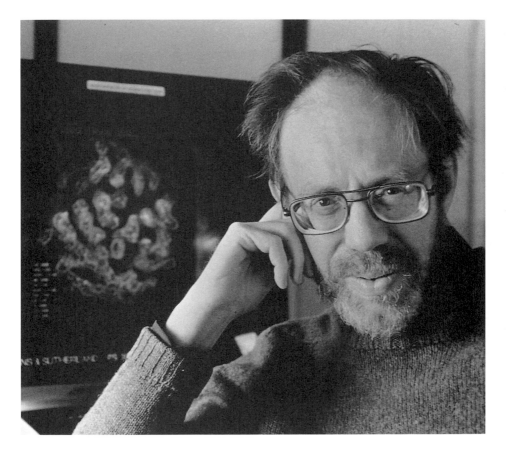

Michael Rossmann (shown here) along with his colleague, Tom Smith, have been experimenting with drugs called capsid binders that may help to stop cold viruses. A computer model of the rhinovirus is shown in the background.

canyon floor. Like the hollow in a rubber ball, the cavities allow the virus to be more flexible. When the drugs fill the cavities, they keep the virus rigid and lock its surface so that it can't open up and let its genetic material free inside the target cell. Thus the viral nucleic acid is unable to direct the production of new virus particles to infect additional cells. Other drug companies have created capsid binders that work on a wider range of cold viruses.

"Since many viruses seem to have basically the same structure, maybe we can use the same target in other viruses. HIV, the AIDS virus, for example, may have a pocket like this. If we find it, then we can try to design drugs that will fit into it," says Dr. Rossman.[3]

Unfortunately, a major problem for capsid binding may be that the viruses can build up resistance to drugs of this type. A single change in the amino acid structure at the bottom of the virus canyon could prevent the drug from binding there. When viruses multiply, both exact and inexact copies are created, yielding various mutant forms. Dr. Margaret Johnson-Lussenburg of the University of Ottawa, points out that the tendency of the virus to mutate might actually help in a drug's effectiveness, if the drug were like a skeleton key that fit as many strains as possible.[4]

By focusing on stopping the virus before it gets into a cell, researchers don't have to worry about the problem of resistance. "It's an absolute requirement that the virus bind to a receptor in order to get into a cell. It would be virtually impossible for the virus to sidestep that receptor and develop

HARD TIMES FOR COLD RESEARCH

Economic times have hurt common cold research. In 1972 the National Institutes of Health abandoned the hunt for a vaccine against the two hundred viruses that cause colds, and federal support was greatly reduced. Much of the recent research in the field has been done in association with pharmaceutical companies.

Cold researchers suffered another blow in 1990 when the world's first cold research center was closed. Each year since 1946, the British government had paid for hundreds of men and women to stay at the Common Cold Research Unit center for ten-day periods to try to catch colds. Some couples even met and fell in love there! The Common Cold Unit made it possible to study large groups of men and women of different ages at a reasonable cost. Over a thousand clinical studies were conducted at the unit before it was closed.

Cold research still continues at other places, such as the University of Virginia, which provides $350 pay and free accommodations for volunteers. The studies, however, are focused mainly on drug trials.[3]

resistance," says Dr. Michael Kamaract, vice president for research at Molecular Therapeutics, part of the Miles Research Center in New Haven, Connecticut.[6] If the viruses mutate so that they don't attach to receptors "they're dead viruses," adds Dr. Steven D. Marlin of Boehringer-Ingelheim Pharmaceuticals in Ridgefield, Connecticut.[7]

Blocking Rhinovirus Receptors

In 1982 Richard Colonno, working at Merck Sharp & Dohme Research Laboratories, began trying to find a way to block cellular receptors so that viruses cannot attach to them. When he tested twenty-four different rhinoviruses, he found that twenty of them attached to the same receptor. From this he was able to calculate that nearly 90 percent of rhinoviruses would attach to that receptor.

Dr. Colonno had not identified where the receptor actually was, but after thousands of experimental tests he discovered an antibody that can attach to the receptor. Working with Jack Gwaltney and Fred Hayden at the University of Virginia, Dr. Colonno tested his theory that spraying the antibody into the noses of healthy volunteers would prevent them from getting colds. Although most of the volunteers came down with colds, "the people treated with the antibodies developed symptoms one to two days later than those in the untreated group," and "their symptoms were only half as severe," says Colonno.[8] Now working at Bristol-Myers Squibb, he is trying to find smaller drug molecules that will block the cell's rhinovirus receptor, without themselves provoking a reaction by the immune system.

In 1989 two different research teams independently identified the cellular receptor that 90 percent of rhinoviruses use to get into nasal cells. It turned out to be a part of the body's immune system: a molecule that binds lymphocytes during their fight against infection. The researchers named this "sticky" molecule intercellular adhesion molecule-1 (ICAM-1). This receptor plays two roles in viral infection. It marks the place for virus particles to attach, and it also helps the virus to shed its outer coat so that it can infect the cell. Antibodies directed against ICAM-1 prevent cells from being infected, apparently by covering up the receptor so that the virus cannot interact with it.

Making a Virus Decoy

Once the cellular receptor had been identified, researchers were able to try another approach to stop cold viruses. Large numbers of genetically engineered ICAM-1 molecules, sprayed into the nose, could act as a decoy to bind rhinoviruses and keep them away from nasal cells. Miles Research Lab and Boehringer-Ingelheim are both testing ICAM nasal sprays and have had promising results in test-tube studies.

Dr. Arnold Monto of the University of Michigan points out that ICAM-1 blockers and capsid binders will not be perfect solutions. Antivirals will not remain in the nose very long because mucus and ciliary action clear particles from the nose fairly quickly. Moreover, both drugs work on rhinoviruses, which cause only 30 to 50 percent of common colds. They wouldn't work on colds caused by the nearly one hundred other cold viruses.[9]

Other Avenues

Other researchers are exploring better cold remedies, believing that the only hope of "curing" the cold will be to relieve symptoms. In 1992, for example, Dr. Steven J. Sperber and colleagues at the University of Virginia announced that a drug called naproxen, which is used for arthritis and menstrual pain, was effective at relieving major cold symptoms such as headache, tiredness, muscle ache, and cough.[10]

Researchers at Nova Pharmaceuticals in Baltimore are testing bradykinin antagonists, substances that block the receptors in nasal tissue for bradykinins, proteins that stimulate inflammation. As many as fifty other substances are involved in the inflammatory reactions that produce the uncomfortable symptoms of a cold. Some of these may also be points of attack for better cold remedies.

A Cold Vaccine?

In 1972 the U.S. government gave up on the hope of ever finding a cold vaccine, and many scientists agreed. There are just too many viruses that cause colds. But some scientists think that cold vaccines may still be possible.

Recent studies have found that most colds in any given region are caused by a particular type of virus, and that the virus remains in the area for a while. This may mean that vaccines for specific types of colds can be given in a specific region to prevent them from spreading further.

Roland Rueckert at the University of Wisconsin in Madison is using genetic engineering to produce monoclonal antibodies—very pure antibodies to rhinoviruses. His team is trying to find common denominators that many cold viruses share, which may cause antibodies to be produced against a large number of rhinoviruses. Someday scientists may have a vaccine that can be sprayed into the nose to trigger antibody protection against most cold-causing viruses.

At Rutgers University in New Brunswick, New Jersey, researchers led by Edward Arnold are experimenting with forcing cold viruses to alter their structure so that antibodies will be able to recognize them more easily. Rhinoviruses are so successful in continuing to infect people because they trick the immune system. Four regions on the virus surface tend to mutate rapidly, constantly producing new loop-shaped structures. Each time a change occurs, the body's immune system learns to recognize the new antigens and makes antibodies to them. But most of this effort is wasted because the loops change again before the antibodies have a chance to work.

The Rutgers researchers are using genetic engineering to make new viruses in which the constantly changing loops are replaced by less mutable amino acid sequences. Using cold virus strains that do not produce symptoms, Arnold's group has incorporated antigens from polio, influenza, and AIDS viruses, producing vaccines that may give protection from these diseases. The researchers believe that they can use the same principle to make cold viruses, by splicing portions of virus structure that do not change very often onto the surface of suitable rhinoviruses.[11]

Flu Vaccines

We have been successfully fighting influenza with vaccines since the 1940s. But researchers are still working to make better flu vaccines—ones that can protect people against more flue virus strains and do so without producing unpleasant side effects.

At the New York State Department of Health researchers have inserted genes from an influenza virus into the cowpox virus, which is very large. (This is the virus that was used to produce the first vaccine against smallpox.) When animals are given the hybrid cowpox vaccine, the immune system produces antibodies to the flu. If people were inoculated with this type of vaccine, there would be no risk of getting the flu because flu viruses are not present. And the cowpox virus is so large that several different strains of flu viruses could fit into the vaccine together.

Another vaccine uses "live" flu viruses. Researchers breed a virus that can function only in low temperatures. When the virus gets into the warm human body, it will not be able to infect cells. Then the harmless virus is crossbred with an infectious influenza virus. The resulting hybrid is still harmless but carries the identifying H and N spikes of the currently circulating flu strain. Antibodies produced against the vaccine virus will thus protect people from the infectious strains. In experiments researchers have found this "live" virus to be more effective then "killed" vaccines against influenza A.[12]

In 1992 researchers at Johns Hopkins University in Baltimore announced a new nose-drop flu vaccine that was effective for preventing influenza A in infants two to five months old. Children younger than six months are not usually given standard flu vaccines because they sometimes cause fever in infants and often do not protect them from the flu virus. According to researcher Dr. Mark C. Steinhoff, "Giving infants the vaccine through the nose is very safe. We have not seen any fever complications, and the children make sufficient antibodies."[13] The new vaccine was also effective for adults. The nose-drop flu vaccine may also bring immunity earlier than a standard vaccine because it stimulates antibody production in the nose where antibodies are needed.

In 1993 a major new advance was announced by researchers from Vical, a new biotechnology company, and Merck Research Laboratories in West Point, Pennsylvania. Genes for a protein inside the flu virus, when injected into the muscles of mice, prompted the production of antibodies against the flu protein. The mice then were able to survive exposure to lethal doses of flu virus. An exciting aspect of the experiment is the fact that the virus used to challenge the immunized mice was an entirely different strain from the one whose genes were injected. This cross-strain protection was possible because the protein inside the flu virus does not tend to mutate the way the surface antigens do.[14]

Antiviral Drugs

The antiviral drug amantadine is now being used to protect high-risk people during flu epidemics. (The related drug rimantadine was approved in 1993 for use in the United States.) But sometimes flu viruses become resistant to these antiviral drugs.

Researchers have identified the flu virus gene that is responsible for amantadine and rimantadine resistance, and they have already decoded portions of the gene that undergo changes during mutation. Eventually this finding may help researchers better understand how the influenza virus reproduces, which would in turn help them develop more effective ways to block the spread of the virus. Basic research like these studies and those that revealed how cold viruses enter nasal cells offer the best hope for new weapons in our fight against the common cold and the flu.

Q&A

Q. Will I catch a cold if I go outside in the winter with my hair wet?

A. Maybe, but only if you have been exposed to a cold virus. Getting chilled might stress your body and lower your resistance, making it easier to catch a cold if you have been exposed to the virus. However, some studies suggest that getting wet and chilled may not make much difference.

Q. Why do I keep catching cold? I thought people developed immunity to disease that they've had already.

A. They do, but there are at least 200 different cold viruses, and each one is able to mutate, changing its surface so that your antibodies won't recognize it anymore. And immunity to colds lasts only a few years, not for a lifetime.

Q. I was supposed to go to visit my grandmother, but when she heard I had a cold she told me not to come. Wasn't she overreacting? It was only a cold!

A. Perhaps, but as a person gets older the immune system works less efficiently, and many elderly people have chronic health problems such as heart disease or respiratory difficulties. They are more likely to develop complications, which might become serious or even life-threatening.

Q. Why do I get a cold every time I go back to school in the fall? Is it the weather?

A. More likely it is because you are in close contact with a lot of people in closed-in classrooms, and catch their cold viruses.

Q. I had a bad chest cold for two weeks. Then the doctor gave me an antibiotic, and I felt a lot better the next day. I thought antibiotics didn't work on colds.

A. The fact that your symptoms lasted so long and affected your chest suggests that you had caught a secondary bacterial infection in your lungs after the original cold weakened your body defenses.

Q. Can I avoid colds and flu by taking extra vitamin C?

A. Vitamin C does help to strengthen the body's immune system and thus may boost your defenses against colds and other infectious diseases. But doctors are still debating whether "megadoses" of vitamin C can prevent colds. Some studies indicate that taking vitamin C can make cold symptoms milder if you do catch a cold.

Q. Why do I catch a cold every year in May or June? Each time, I am sneezing and blowing my nose for more than a month.

A. When respiratory symptoms recur each year around the same time of year, they are most likely from an allergy rather than a cold. There is a wave of "hay fever" outbreaks in the early spring caused by allergies to tree pollens and another in the early summer due to grass pollens; many people suffer from ragweed pollen allergies from mid-August through September. "Winter colds" may actually be allergies to molds or dust mites.

Q. Should I take aspirin for the fever and aches of the flu?

A. Fever is part of the body's defense against viruses, but a very high fever can be dangerous. Anyone under eighteen should take acetaminophen for a fever caused by a viral infection because taking aspirin might produce the dangerous Reye's syndrome.

Q. Should I go to the doctor if I have a cold or flu?

A. You should see a doctor if a fever lasts for more than two days, if a cold or flu lasts more than a week, if a cough is keeping you from sleeping, and if chest symptoms, severe headache, stiff neck, or other complications develop.

Q. Why is flu more dangerous than a cold?

A. The flu virus destroys more cells in the lining of the respiratory tract and produces severer symptoms. The virus can also invade the lungs, resulting in pneumonia, and flu is more likely to lead to secondary bacterial infections that may be life-threatening.

Cold and Flu Timeline

500 B.C.—Hippocrates said colds were caused by waste matter in the brain.

1600s—Italians called the flu *influenza*.

1700s—Benjamin Franklin said colds were spread from person to person.

1898 —Martinus Willem Beijerinck showed the existence of viruses.

1914 —Walter von Kruse suggested that viruses cause colds.

1918 —Spanish flu pandemic swept the world.

1931 —Pathologist Richard Shope proved swine flu was caused by a virus.

1933 —Influenza type A virus identified.

1938 —Alphonse R. Dochez confirmed viral cause of colds.

1940 —Influenza type B virus identified.

1941 —Wade H. Frost concluded that there are many cold viruses.

1947 —Influenza type C virus identified.

1955 —Sir Christopher Andrewes identified the first cold virus.

1957 —Asian flu pandemic swept the world.

1968 —Hong Kong flu pandemic swept the world.

1978 —Marvin Sackner established that chicken soup clears congestion.

1985 —Michael Rossmann demonstrated the 3-D structure of a cold virus.

For More Information

American Lung Association
1740 Broadway
New York, NY 10019
(212) 315-8700
(Your local branch may be listed in
your local telephone directory.)

Centers for Disease Control
1600 Clifton Road, NE
Atlanta, GA 30333
(404) 332-4555
(Influenza Helpline, identifies flu
strains and outbreaks around the
United States.)

**National Jewish Center for Immunology
and Respiratory Medicine**
1400 Jackson Street
Denver, CO 80206
(800) 222-LUNG
(Lung Line, provides free advice
about respiratory illness.)

Chapter Notes

Chapter 1

1. Wendy Murphy, *Coping with the Common Cold* (Alexandria, Va.: Time-Life Books, 1981), pp. 6, 8.

2. "Uncommon ICAM Blocks Common Cold Virus," *Science News* (March 10, 1990), p. 156.

3. Stephanie Scott, "The Common Cold," *Vim & Vigor* (Winter 1991), p. 24.

4. Jeffrey P. Cohn, "Here Come the Bugs," *FDA Consumer* (November 1988), p. 6.

5. *The Common Cold,* National Institute of Allergy and Infectious Diseases, Bethesda, Md. (1988 booklet).

6. Joanne Silberner, "Best Ways to Fight the Cold," *U.S. News & World Report* (January 29, 1990), p. 54.

7. Washington Post Wire Service, "Flu Diagnosis Covers Multitude of Woes," *The Star-Ledger* (Newark, N.J.) (January 19, 1992), p. H3.

Chapter 2

1. Wendy Murphy, *Coping with the Common Cold* (Alexandria, Va.: Time-Life Books, 1981), pp. 101–102.

2. Charles Clayman, ed., *The American Medical Association: Encyclopedia of Medicine* (New York: Random House, 1989) p. 287; Patricia Thomas, "Common Colds," *Medical World News* (April 1991), p. 24; Joanne Silberner, "Best Ways to Fight That Cold," *U.S. News & World Report* (January 29, 1990), p. 54.

3. Ibid., p. 9.

4. Mary Kittredge, *The Common Cold* (New York: Chelsea House, 1989), p. 52.

5. Peter Jaret, "It All Starts With a Sneeze," *Health* (November, 1988), p. 55.

6. Stephanie Scott, "The Common Cold," *Vim & Vigor* (Winter 1991), p. 23.

7. Kittredge, p. 14.

Chapter 3

1. Associated Press, "Clinton Challenges GOP for Better Idea," *The Courier News* (Bridgewater, N.J.) (February 21, 1993), p. A9.

2. Jeffrey P. Cohn, "Here Come the Bugs," *FDA Consumer* (November 1988), p. 6.

3. Patricia Thomas, "Common Colds," *Medical World News* (April, 1991), p. 29.

4. Stephanie Scott, "The Common Cold," *Vim & Vigor* (Winter 1991), p. 24.

5. Ibid.

6. Nancy Stedman, *The Common Cold and Influenza* (New York: Julian Messner, 1986), p. 19.

7. Peter Jaret, "It All Starts With a Sneeze," *Health* (November, 1988), p. 55.

8. Mary Kittredge, *The Common Cold* (New York: Chelsea House, 1989), p. 31; Wendy Murphy, *Coping with the Common Cold (Alexandria, Va.: Time-Life Books, 1981), p. 17.*

9. Patricia Thomas, "Common Misery," *Harvard Health Letter* (November, 1991), p. 7.

10. Ibid.

Chapter 4

1. Mary Roach, "How I Blew My Summer Vacation," *In Health* (January/February 1990), pp. 73–80.

2. Chris Anne Raymond, "Fighting the Common Cold," *World Book Health & Medical Annual, 1987)* , p. 46.

3. Joanne Silberner, "Best Ways to Fight that Cold," *U.S. News and World Report* (January 29, 1990), p. 56.

4. Patricia Thomas, "Common Misery," *Harvard Health Letter* (November, 1991), p. 7.

5. Raymond, p. 46.

6. Peter Jaret, "It All Starts With a Sneeze," *Health* (November, 1988), p. 56.

7. Thomas, "Common Misery," p. 8.

8. Peggy Rynk, "Natural Cold Remedies," *Let's Live* (December, 1990), p. 28.

9. Mary Kittredge, *The Common Cold (New York: Chelsea House, 1989), p. 50.*

10. Silberner, p. 60.

11. Patricia Thomas, "Common Colds," *Medical World News* (April, 1991), p. 29.

12. "Prevention and Treatment of the Common Cold," *Pharmacy Times* (July 1988), p. 101.

13. Wendy Murphy, *Coping with the Common Cold,* (Alexandria, Va.: Time-Life Books, 1981), p. 11.

14. Los Angeles Times, "Study Says Flu, Stress Are Linked," *The Courier News* (Bridgewater, N.J.) (August 29, 1991), p. A-10.

Chapter 5

1. Patricia Thomas, "Common Colds," *Medical World News* (April, 1991), p. 24.

2. Eran Esar, ed., *The Dictionary of Humorous Quotations* (New York: Dorset Press, 1989), p. 102.

3. Patricia Thomas, "Cold Comforts," *Harvard Health Letter* (December 1991), p. 5.

4. Stephanie Scott, "The Common Cold," *Vim & Vigor* (Winter 1991), p. 25.

5. "The Cold," booklet from Sandoz Pharmaceuticals, East Hanover, N.J., dated 1989.

6. Thomas, "Cold Comforts," p. 5.

7. ". . . Drinking Milk," *Bottom Line* (January 30, 1991), p. 9.

8. Steven Findlay, "The Experts' Cures: Hot Showers, Straight Gin," *U.S. News & World Report* (January 29, 1990), p. 59.

9. Judith J. Wurtman, "Cold War and You," *Bottom Line* (February 15, 1992), p. 10.

10. Stephen Edgington, "Biotechnology and the Common Cold," *Bio/Technology* (May 1992), p. 502.

11. Thomas, "Cold Comforts," p. 6.

12. Ibid.

13. Scott, p. 26.

14. "Value of Cold Remedies Challenged," *The New York Times* (September 14, 1991), p. C11.

15. Thomas, "Cold Comforts," p. 5.

16. D. A. J. Tyrrell, "Common Cold," *Britannica Medical & Health Annual, 1991,* p. 260.

17. "Steam Cure for Colds: Full of Hot Air?" *Science News* (September 1,1990) p.141.

18. "Zinc and Colds," *The New York Times* (October 14, 1992), p. C14.

19. Clark Norton, "The Purple Coneflower's Comeback," *Health* (September 1992), pp. 26–28.

Chapter 6

1. Jean Carper, "Study Suggests Daily Intake of Yogurt Bolsters Fight Against the Common Cold," *The Star-Ledger* (Newark, N.J.) (October 21, 1992), p. 70.

2. Mary Kittredge, *The Common Cold* (New York: Chelsea House, 1989), p. 78.

3. Ibid., p. 77–78.

4. Linus Pauling, *Vitamin C and the Common Cold* (San Francisco: W. H. Freeman, 1970), p. 52.

5. Nancy Stedman, *The Common Cold and Influenza (New York: Julian Messner, 1986), p. 49.*

6. Wendy Murphy, *Coping with the Common Cold (Alexandria, Va.: Time-Life Books, 1981), p. 146.*

7. Patricia Thomas, "Common Colds," *Medical World News* (April, 1991), p. 30.

8. Patricia Thomas, "Cold Comforts," *Harvard Health Letter* (December, 1991), p. 6.

9. Thomas, "Common Colds," p. 30.

10. Patricia Thomas, "Interferon Gets Second Try After '80s Flop," *Medical World News* (April, 1991), p. 27.

11. Stephen Edgington, "Biotechnology and the Common Cold," *Bio/Technology* (May 1992), p. 507; Anita Cecchin, "Cold Comfort," *Medical World News* (March, 1993), p. 38.

12. Murphy, p. 41.

13. Stephanie Scott, "The Common Cold," *Vim & Vigor* (Winter 1991), p. 27; "The Common Cold," *Drug Topics* (December 10, 1990), p. 37.

14. Thomas, "Common Colds," p. 29.

15. Kittredge, p. 16.

Chapter 7

1. Wendy Murphy, *Coping with the Common Cold (Alexandria, Va.: Time-Life Books, 1981), p. 104.*

2. Nancy Stedman, *The Common Cold and Influenza (New York, Julian Messner, 1986), p. 38.*

3. Jack Fincher, "America's Deadly Rendezvous With the 'Spanish Lady,'" *Smithsonian* (January 1989) pp. 131–145.

4. Richard Trubo, "Down and Out With the Flu," *The World Book Health & Medical Annual 1993*, p. 142.

5. Nancy H. Arden, "Flu," *Britannica Medical & Health Annual, 1991*, p. 419.

6. David White and Frank Fenner, *Medical Virology* (New York: Academic Press, 1986), p. 515.

7. Jeffrey Cohn, "Here Come the Bugs," *FDA Consumer* (November, 1988), p. 6.

8. Arden, p. 418.

9. Bernice Kanner, "Cold Wars," *New York* (September 30, 1991), p. 12.

10. Washington Post Wire Service, "Flu Diagnosis Covers Multitude of Woes," *The Star-Ledger* (Newark, N.J.) (January 19, 1992), p. H3.

11. Catherine O'Neill, "20 Questions to Ask Before You Catch a Cold," *McCall's* (February 1990), p. 84.

12. Ron Gasbarro, "Vaccine and Other Measures Can Take a Big Bite out of the Flu Bug," *The Star-Ledger* (Newark, N.J.) (January 20, 1992), p. 17.

13. Cohn, p. 10.

14. Melinda Beck, "Feeling Bad, Getting Worse," *Newsweek* (February 5, 1990), p. 57.

Chapter 8

1. "Ann Landers" column, *The Courier News* (Bridgewater, N.J.) (November 18, 1992), p. D4.

2. Stephanie Scott, "The Common Cold," *Vim & Vigor* (Winter, 1991), p. 27.

3. Ibid.

4. Stephen Edgington, "Biotechnology and the Common Cold," *Bio/Technology* (May, 1992), p. 504.

5. Ibid, p. 502.

6. Wendy Murphy, *Coping with the Common Cold* (Alexandria, Va.: Time-Life Books, 1981), p. 119.

7. Ibid, p. 122.

Chapter 9

1. Steven Findlay, "Slowly, A Cure Begins To Take Shape," *U.S. News & World Report* (January 29, 1990), p. 58.

2. Peter Radetsky, "Taming the Wily Rhinovirus," *Discover* (April, 1989), p. 43.

3. Radetsky, p. 41.

4. Patricia Thomas, "Common Colds," *Medical World News* (April, 1991), p. 25–26.

5. Mary Roach, "How I Blew My Summer Vacation," *In Health* (January/February, 1990), p. 80; Anita Cecchin, "Government Not Coughing Up the Money for Cold Research," *Medical World News* (March 1993), p. 32.

6. Ibid, p. 26.

7. "Uncommon ICAM Blocks Common Cold Virus," *Science News* (March 10, 1990), p. 156.

8. Radetsky, p. 43.

9. Thomas, p. 26.

10. "Drug Relieves Cold Symptoms," *Healthfacts* (July 1992), p. 1.

11. Stephen Edgington, "Biotechnology and the Common Cold," *Bio/Technology* (May, 1992), pp. 504–505.

12. Nancy Stedman, *The Common Cold and Influenza (New York: Julian Messner, 1986), p. 54.*

13. Andrea Kott, "Nose-drop Flu Vaccine is Effective in Infants," *Medical Tribune* (May 21, 1992), p. 3.

14. Jon Cohen, "Naked DNA Points Way to Vaccines," *Science* (March 19, 1993), pp. 1691–1692.

Glossary

adenoids—Masses of lymphoid tissue in the upper respiratory passages.

adenoviruses—A group of cold-causing viruses.

aerosol—A suspension of liquid droplets in the air.

amantadine—An antiviral drug effective against flu.

antibodies—Proteins produced to bind specifically to foreign chemicals (*antigens*), such as surface chemicals on an invading virus.

antigenic drift—A gradual change in a virus due to the accumulation of small genetic changes *(mutations)*.

antigenic shift—A sudden, dramatic change in a circulating virus.

antihistamine—A medication to counteract the effects of histamine.

anti-inflammatory—A medication to reduce inflammation.

bradykinin—A chemical secreted by cells, which produces inflammation.

bronchitis—Infection of the larger air passages in the lungs.

communicable disease—One that is spread from one person to another.

cilia—Tiny hairlike structures on the cells in the membrane lining the respiratory passages; they beat back and forth to create an upward current in the mucus.

cough suppressant—A medication that works on the cough center in the brain to prevent coughing.

congestion—A narrowing of the nasal passages due to inflammation of mucous membrane cells in the nasal lining.

coronaviruses—A group of cold-causing viruses.

decongestant—A medication that reduces nasal stuffiness by shrinking blood vessels in the nose.

ephedra—A natural decongestant chemical found in herbs such as mahuang.

epidemic—An infectious disease that spreads over a wide area.

expectorant—A medication that loosens mucus so that it can be coughed up more readily.

hemagglutinin—A surface protein on the flu virus that combines with red blood cells and causes them to clump together.

histamine—A chemical secreted by cells that produces inflammation.

humidifier—A device that adds moisture to the air.

ICAM-1 (intercellular adhesion molecule-1)—The cell receptor used by rhinoviruses to invade nasal cells.

immune system—Various body defenses against invading microbes, including white blood cells and interferon.

immunoglobulin—A blood fraction containing antibodies against disease microbes.

incubation period—The time between infection and appearance of symptoms.

inflammation—Swelling, pain, heat, and redness in the tissues around a site of infection.

interferon—A protein released by virus-infected cells that protects other cells from infection.

laryngitis—Infection of the voice box (*larynx*), producing hoarseness or inability to produce speech sounds.

lymphocytes—Disease-fighting white blood cells that recognize invading microbes and attack them, either directly or by producing antibodies.

macrophages—Disease-fighting white blood cells that engulf microbes.

mucus—A sticky fluid secreted by cells in the membrane lining the respiratory passages.

neuraminidase—A surface protein on the flu virus that helps in the entry of the virus into cells and the release of viruses from infected cells.

neutrophils—Disease-fighting white blood cells that engulf microbes.

orthomyxoviruses—The family of viruses that cause influenza.

otitis—An ear infection.

pandemic—An infectious disease that spreads all around the world, involving millions of people.

pharyngitis—Inflammation of the upper throat (*pharynx*).

pneumonia—A serious illness with sharp chest pain, severe cough, and very high fever, due to infection of lung tissue by viruses or bacteria.

receptor—A specific structure on the cell membrane to which a virus, hormone, or some other active substance attaches.

rhinovirus—A group of viruses responsible for the majority of colds.

rhinitis—Inflammation of the nose.

sinusitis—Infection of the *sinuses* (air-filled spaces in the skull bones, around the eyes and nose).

tonsillitis—Infection of the *tonsils* (masses of lymphoid tissue in the throat that contain disease-fighting white blood cells).

viral shedding—Release of viruses from the body of an infected person.

Further Reading

Books:

Kittredge, Mary. *The Common Cold.* New York: Chelsea House Publishers, 1989.

Murphy, Wendy. *Coping with the Common Cold.* Alexandria, Va.: Time-Life Books, 1981.

Radetsky, Peter. *The Invisible Invaders: The Story of the Emerging Age of Viruses.* Boston: Little, Brown, 1991.

Stedman, Nancy. *The Common Cold and Influenza.* New York: Julian Messner, 1986.

Articles:

Ackerman, S. J. "Flu Shots: Do You Need One?" *FDA Consumer,* October 1989, pp. 8–10.

Arden, Nancy H. "Influenza." *Encyclopaedia Britannica Medical & Health Annual, 1993,* pp. 325–331.

Cecchin, Anita. "Cold Comfort." *Medical World News,* March 1993, pp. 30–42.

Cohen, Jon. "Naked DNA Points Way to Vaccines." *Science,* March 19, 1993, pp. 1691–1692.

Cohn, Jeffrey P. "Here Come the Bugs." *FDA Consumer,* November 1988, pp. 6–13.

Edgington, Stephen M. "Bauhaus Biology: Biotechnology and the Common Cold." *Bio/Technology,* May 1992, pp. 502–507.

Fincher, Jack. "America's Deadly Rendezvous with the 'Spanish Lady.'" *Smithsonian,* January 1989, pp. 131–145.

Henig, Robin Marantz. "Flu Pandemic." *New York Times Magazine,* November 29, 1992, pp. 28–31, 55, 64–67.

Jaret, Peter. "It All Starts With a Sneeze." *Health,* November 1988, pp. 55–57, 84.

Radetsky, Peter. "Taming the Wily Rhinovirus." *Discover,* April 1989, pp. 38–43.

Raymond, Chris Anne. "Fighting the Common Cold." *World Book Health Annual, 1987,* pp. 433–455.

Roach, Mary. "How I Blew My Summer Vacation." *In Health,* January/February 1990, pp. 73–80.

Scott, Stephanie. "The Common Cold." *Vim & Vigor,* Winter 1991, pp. 23–27.

Silberner, Joanne. "Best Ways to Fight That Cold." *U.S. News & World Report,* January 29, 1990, pp. 54–60.

Thomas, Patricia. "Cold Comforts." *Harvard Health Letter,* December 1991, pp. 5–7.

———. "Common Colds: Finally Getting Their Scientific Due." *Medical World News,* April 1991, pp. 24–30.

Trubo, Richard. "Down-and-Out With the Flu." *The World Book Health & Medical Annual, 1993,* pp. 141–153.

Tyrrel, D. A. J. "Common Cold." *Encyclopaedia Britannica Medical & Health Annual, 1991,* pp. 258–260.

Index

127